Basic Lymphoedema Management

Treatment and Prevention of Problems Associated with Lymphatic Filariasis

Gerusa Dreyer, MD
Non-Governmental Organization Amaury Coutinho
– Recife, Brazil

Núcleo de Ensino, Pesquisa e Assistência em Filariose
– NEPAF – Federal University of Pernambuco – Brazil

David Addiss, MD, MPH
Centers for Disease Control and Prevention
– Atlanta, USA

Patricia Dreyer, MD
Non-Governmental Organization Amaury Coutinho
– Recife, Brazil

Joaquim Norões, MD
Núcleo de Ensino, Pesquisa e Assistência em Filariose
– NEPAF – Federal University of Pernambuco – Brazil

Non-Governmental Organization Amaury Coutinho
– Recife, Brazil

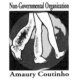

Non-Governmental Organization
Amaury Coutinho

HDI
HEALTH & DEVELOPMENT INTERNATIONAL

ISBN 1-884186-17-3

Hollis Publishing Company
95 Runnells Bridge Road, Hollis, NH 03049
(t) 603.889.4500   (f) 603.889.6551
HOLLIS   books@hollispublishing.com
PUBLISHING

Printed in the United States of America.

♻ Printed on recycled paper.

TABLE OF CONTENTS

CHAPTER ONE

Community Treatment for Lymphatic Filariasis 1

Eliminating Lymphatic Filariasis
Adverse Drug Reactions
Medication for People with Microfilariae in Their Blood

CHAPTER TWO

Filariasis and the Lymphatic Vessels 7

The Lymphatic System
Adult Filarial Worms Damage the Lymphatic Vessels
Consequences of Damaged Lymphatic Vessels Draining the Skin
Consequences of Damaged Lymphatic Vessels Draining Sites Other Than the Skin
Filariasis and the Lymphatic System in Children

CHAPTER THREE

Assessment of Chronic Lymphoedema 13

CHAPTER FOUR

Lymphoedema Management 23

The Need for Lymphoedema Management
The Basic Components of Lymphoedema Management
Steps in Lymphoedema Management

CHAPTER FIVE

Assessment and Management of Acute Attacks 47

Acute Attack Assessment
Acute Attack Management

CHAPTER SIX

Urogenital Problems in Filariasis 53

Genital Problems
Hydrocoele
Problems Affecting the Skin of the Scrotum and Penis
Urinary Tract Problems

CHAPTER SEVEN

**Factors That Complicate Lymphoedema Management
in Filariasis-Endemic Areas** 67

Diseases of the Veins: Venous Insufficiency and Venous Ulcer
Diabetes (High Levels of Blood Sugar)
Psoriasis
Leprosy
Myiasis
Pregnancy
Occlusive and Semi-occlusive Dressings

CHAPTER EIGHT

Differential Diagnosis 73

Swelling of Limbs
Swelling of the Genitals and Breast
Lipedema
Knobs
Milky Urine
Inguinal Hernia

CHAPTER NINE

Achieving, Maintaining, and Monitoring Lymphoedema Programs 79

Achieving Success
Maintaining Success
Hope Clubs
Addressing Challenges
Community Resources
Benefits of Successful Lymphoedema Management
Monitoring Success
Final Words

APPENDIX 89–90

GLOSSARY 91

INDEX 101

RESOURCE INFORMATION 111

FOREWORD

What a treat it will be for those who face the vexing problem of managing lymphoedema and its complications to find this volume! Surely it will become for them a constant and trusted companion, filling a void all too apparent both to those who suffer from lymphoedema disorders and to those who help to manage these disorders. Indeed, it is easy to recognize that *Basic Lymphoedema Management* is anything but a re-hash of older textbook material or patient manuals; it is truly a work 'built from the ground up' and based on the authors' personal observations of literally tens of thousands of individuals in their care.

While it certainly cannot be said that there were not important advances in understanding lymphoedema and its consequences before Dr. Dreyer and her colleagues began their clinical research work in Recife, Brazil during the 1980s, it also cannot be denied that the efforts of this team have absolutely transformed both our thinking and clinical approach to managing lymphatic disorders. Both the clinical essence of that transformed thinking and the patient management recommendations distilled from it are captured very effectively in *Basic Lymphoedema Management*, but it is also important for the reader to know that there is an equally impressive body of basic knowledge amassed by this same research team that, in fact, serves as the scientific underpinning for all of the clinical observations, interpretations and recommendations found in this volume.

Far and away the most common cause of the severe lymphoedema disorders worldwide is infection with lymphatic filarial parasites (*Wuchereria bancrofti, Brugia malayi* and *B. timori*) which affect an estimated 120 million persons and put more than a billion people at risk of infection. Remarkable research advances of the past two decades have given us treatment tools and strategies now effective enough to contemplate interrupting transmission of this mosquito-borne infection and even to lead the World Health Assembly in 1997 to call for the elimination of lymphatic filariasis (LF) as a public health problem worldwide. Generous donations towards this goal by both the private sector (especially GlaxoSmithKline and Merck & Co., Inc.) and the public sector have enabled the creation of a Global Alliance to Eliminate Lymphatic Filariasis that now supports active national LF-elimination programs in almost half of the world's 80 endemic countries.

The success of these efforts to stop the spread of filarial infection will *prevent* new cases of lymphatic damage and its clinical consequences, but the enormous challenge of helping—i.e., alleviating the suffering and preventing disability—those already with damaged lymphatics and clinical disease must still be faced. What tools are available to meet this challenge? Principally those defined by Dr. Dreyer, her co-authors and collaborators around the world—and detailed in this first edition of *Basic Lymphoedema Management*! Indeed, it is these basic concepts of clinical management of filarial disease that have formed the core curriculum for all training activities, first initiated at the International Training Center in Lymphatic Filariasis in Recife, Brazil by the four authors and subsequently disseminated with World Health Organization support throughout the Global Programme to Eliminate Lymphatic Filariasis.

Care for those with filarial disease (lymphoedema, elephantiasis, hydrocoele and other genital damage) does not, however, stop with just technical correctness; it must also address the needs of the 'whole individual' including his or her relationships with family and community. Not only is LF a stigmatizing disease, it also exacts a severe toll on an individual's sense of self-worth and ability to fulfill satisfactorily the expected social, sexual and economic roles in life. Without the prescription for success outlined in this volume, hopelessness was long a hallmark of this chronic disabling disease.

In *Basic Lymphoedema Management* the authors' sense of urgency to share the new understandings about successful management of filarial disease and to equip patients to dispel such emotions of hopelessness can be felt in almost every page. Indeed, it has been this 'whole person' focus of all four authors of this volume that has driven their own research and clinical programs from the outset. These are not authors dispassionate in their clinical approach to patients; rather, it is their passionate concern for the lymphoedema-affected individual that motivates them to dig further and further into the unknown, to find solutions for both the complex medical and the 'simple life' problems brought on by lymphatic filarial disease, and to imbue in their patients a *realism* of hope and self-worth that comes with proper attentiveness to self-care and to the life-long principles of self-management.

Basic Lymphoedema Management brings together the practical, clinical conclusions culminating from decades of clinical and research observations by its four authors in Recife and elsewhere. It will be a treasure for those managing filarial disease as well as for those responsible for developing the strategies and integrating disease management principles into the broader Global Programme to Eliminate Lymphatic Filariasis. But, without question, it will certainly prove to be an even greater treasure for the tens of millions of affected individuals who will benefit directly from the knowledge it imparts. It is for me, therefore, a distinct privilege to be able to introduce, on behalf of its authors, this remarkable volume on *Basic Lymphoedema Management* to the health community and those it serves.

ERIC A. OTTESEN, MD

Lymphatic Filariasis Support Center
Department of International Health
Rollins School of Public Health, Emory University
Atlanta, GA

PREFACE

The human suffering that results from lymphatic filariasis can scarcely be imagined. An estimated 14 million persons suffer from lymphoedema or elephantiasis of the leg and as many as 25 million men have urogenital disease caused by lymphatic filariasis. The obvious effects of these conditions on physical mobility and capacity to work have led the World Health Organization to rank lymphatic filariasis as the second leading cause of long-term disability worldwide. Perhaps even more important, however, are the devastating, but often hidden, psychological and social effects of disfigurement, uncontrolled odour, sexual disability, and painful acute bacterial infections.

This book represents the fruit of more than 18 years of patient care and clinical research. When we began this work, elephantiasis was considered the irreversible endpoint of lymphatic filariasis. Patients had little hope of improvement and most health care providers, feeling equally helpless, provided little in the way of care for these patients.

Recent conceptual and practical advances, derived in large part from clinical observations in Recife, Brazil, and a renewed appreciation of the importance of secondary bacterial infections in progression of lymphoedema and elephantiasis, have provided new hope to patients and health workers alike. In May, 1997, the World Health Assembly passed a resolution calling for "global elimination of lymphatic filariasis as a public health problem." As the Global Programme to Eliminate Lymphatic Filariasis began to develop with the primary goal of preventing filarial infection and disease in future generations, it became clear that the magnitude of human suffering caused by existing filarial disease simply could not be ignored. Thus, "morbidity control," or "disability prevention and rehabilitation," was adopted as the second major pillar of the new program.

This book is intended for health care workers with a moderate level of training and for program managers in filariasis-endemic areas. It is particularly intended for health workers responsible for providing care to persons with lymphoedema and for training others in lymphoedema management. When technical terms are used, they are defined within the text and in a glossary at the end of the book. We hope that this book also is useful for students of nursing, medicine, and allied health fields, as well as for physicians and nurses.

The book is not intended to be a comprehensive reference for the management of lymphoedema in hospitalised patients, or in patients with other medical conditions that may complicate the treatment or confuse the diagnosis of lymphoedema (although some of these conditions are described in Chapter 7). Rather, it is intended for health workers at the local or district level who may not have access to microscopes, bacterial cultures, or other diagnostic tests. Similarly, the focus of this book is limited to the management of lymphoedema in persons living in filariasis-endemic areas, in the context of public health programs to eliminate lymphatic filariasis. The field of lymphology has made great strides during the past two decades, and new lymphoedema treatment modalities, including compressive bandaging, massage, and other components of complex decongestive physiotherapy, have proved highly effective in Europe, Australia, and North America. Although individual patients in filariasis-endemic areas may benefit from some of these more expensive or sophisticated techniques, our focus has remained on the basics of lymphoedema management, which should be available to all patients. Finally, this is not a textbook of lymphatic filariasis or of filariasis elimination; we have provided only limited information on antifilarial drug treatment to introduce the health worker to the relationship between lymphatic filariasis and lymphoedema.

The new seven-stage classification for lymphoedema proposed in this book was developed as part of the effort to eliminate lymphatic filariasis as a public health problem. It is possible that some patients in filariasis-endemic areas will not easily fit into one of the seven stages. In some settings, it may be desirable to collapse or combine certain stages (e.g., stages 1 and 2) for use in epidemiologic surveys, for establishing criteria for decision-making and referral by peripheral health workers, or for other purposes. Further refinement of these criteria may be necessary for optimising care of the individual patient by physicians. The authors welcome suggestions for improvement and revision of these criteria. In addition, we would like to hear about problems in patient management that were not anticipated or addressed.

Even though drugs are now available to interrupt transmission of the filarial parasite, lymphoedema care is a life-long process. The competing demands for survival in many filariasis-endemic areas make long-term maintenance of lymphoedema care a challenge. For most patients, especially those with early-stage disease, lymphoedema care can be incorporated into the daily routine at home, very inexpensively. However, patient motivation is essential, and the health care provider can play an important role in enhancing the patient's commitment to life-long lymphoedema care. He or she can help the patient tremendously by encouraging creative solutions to barriers as they arise.

This book focuses on relieving the physical pain and disability associated with lymphatic filariasis. However, social isolation, mental suffering, and stigmatisation are often more formidable barriers to a dignified life for these patients. The health care provider can be a source of hope and support for these patients by maintaining a positive attitude, showing kindness and concern, and offering words of encouragement.

The evolution of this book has benefited from the hard work and helpful comments of many colleagues, and of students who participated in lymphoedema training courses in Haiti, Brazil, China, India and the Dominican Republic. We would like to thank Julie Bettinger and Dr. Anne Peterson for their valuable contributions to a training manual that was used in these courses; Maude Heurtelou and Mama Blue for enthusiastic encouragement; Dr. Anders Seim and Health & Development International for financial support of the book's publication under a grant for disability prevention and alleviation; GlaxoSmithKline for a travel grant to complete the writing; and NGO Amaury Coutinho, which provided technical and material support. Dr. Eric Ottesen provided the conditions and encouragement that made it possible to finalize this book. Most of all, we are indebted to our patients, who have been our most effective teachers, encouragers, and motivators.

GERUSA DREYER, MD
DAVID ADDISS, MD, MPH

Recife, Brazil

CHAPTER ONE
Community Treatment for Lymphatic Filariasis

As a health care provider, you have seen people in your community who suffer from lymphatic filariasis. More than 120 million men, women and children suffer from this disease and its lasting effects. The World Health Organisation lists lymphatic filariasis as a leading cause of disability worldwide.

Lymphatic filariasis is a disease caused by parasitic worms that are spread from person to person by mosquitoes. When a mosquito takes a human blood meal, the worms are deposited on the surface of the skin; they enter the skin, find their way to the lymphatic vessels, and, during a period of 6 to 12 months, develop into adult worms (Fig. 1.01). The adult worms mate and the females release millions of tiny worms, called microfilariae. Microfilariae live in the blood, and can be seen only with a microscope (Fig. 1.02).

When mosquitoes feed on people who have microfilariae in their blood, they take up the microfilariae in the blood meal. The microfilariae develop inside the mosquito. Within 7 to 10 days, the worms can be spread to other people when the mosquito takes another blood meal. Thus, mosquitoes are required to spread the worms from one person to another (Fig. 1.03).

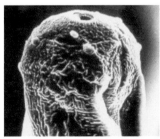

Fig. 1.01 Head of a female adult worm as seen with an electron microscope (courtesy of Dr. A. C. Araújo). Adult filarial worms live in the lymphatic vessels.

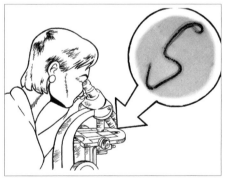

Fig. 1.02 Microfilariae, or tiny worms, are released by the female adult worm and live in the blood. Microfilariae can be seen in a sample of blood only with a microscope.

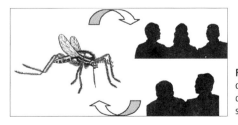

Fig. 1.03 Microfilariae are taken up by mosquitoes during a blood meal. In the mosquito, microfilariae develop into filarial worms that can once again be spread to people.

Two different types of worms can cause lymphatic filariasis in humans. About 90% of infections are caused by the worm *Wuchereria bancrofti*. This type of filariasis, known as bancroftian filariasis, occurs in Africa, Asia, the Pacific Islands, and the Americas. *Brugia malayi*, which occurs in Asia and some Pacific islands, accounts for about 10% of human filariasis. This book was written for health workers in areas with bancroftian filariasis. However, the principles also should be useful for health care providers in areas with brugian filariasis.

Lymphatic filariasis may cause a variety of medical problems. In men with bancroftian filariasis, the most common problem is hydrocoele, or excess fluid inside the scrotal sac (see chapter 6 for more information). People may also have swelling in the legs (Fig. 1.04), arms (Fig. 1.05), breasts (Fig. 1.06), scrotum, and penis (Fig. 1.07). This swelling is called lymphoedema. You may have heard the term elephantiasis, which

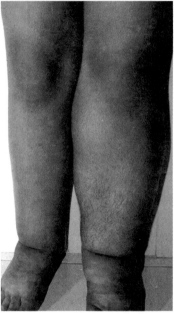

Fig. 1.04   A patient with lymphoedema of the legs.

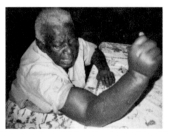

Fig. 1.05   A patient with lymphoedema of the right arm.

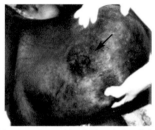

Fig. 1.06   A patient with elephantiasis of the breast. The nipple is indicated by an arrow.

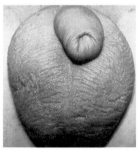

Fig. 1.07   A patient with lymphoedema of the scrotum and penis.

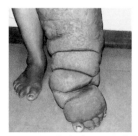

Fig. 1.08   A patient with elephantiasis of the left leg.

refers to the most advanced stages of lymphoedema (Fig. 1.08). *Many people with lymphatic filariasis have no obvious signs of disease, although their lymphatic vessels are already damaged, and they are at risk of developing lymphoedema.*

Neither infection with the filarial worm nor any of the medical problems caused by lymphatic filariasis—hydrocoele, lymphoedema, or elephantiasis, for example—can be spread from one person to another by touching, kissing, sex, or other types of personal contact. Children cannot get hydrocoele or elephantiasis from their parents.

Unlike bancroftian filariasis, brugian filariasis does not affect the genital area. In areas with brugian filariasis, the main medical problem related to lymphatic filariasis is lymphoedema of the legs, which occurs in both men and women.

Eliminating Lymphatic Filariasis

In 1998, the World Health Organisation announced a program to eliminate lymphatic filariasis throughout the world. Drugs are now available that, when taken in a single dose, kill microfilariae and keep the blood free of them for up to a year. This prevents mosquitoes from spreading lymphatic filariasis from one person to another. The drugs that kill the microfilariae do not kill all the adult worms, which live for 5 to 10 years and may continue to produce microfilariae. Therefore, annual treatment to kill microfilariae must be continued for several years.

Two major drugs are available to kill the microfilariae in the blood: diethylcarbamazine (DEC) and ivermectin. A third drug, albendazole, kills other worms that live in the intestine. Albendazole may also make DEC and ivermectin more effective in keeping the blood free of microfilariae. Ivermectin has been donated under the name of Mectizan® (Merck, Inc.) for lymphatic filariasis in many countries in Africa. Albendazole is donated in all filariasis-endemic areas by the drug company GlaxoSmithKline.

Another way to eliminate lymphatic filariasis is for everyone in affected communities to use salt that is fortified with DEC in place of their regular table or cooking salt. This method has been used successfully in China. People who use DEC-fortified salt get a small dose of DEC every day. These small doses are enough to clear the blood of microfilariae and they cause no adverse reactions (see below).

Adverse Drug Reactions

DEC, ivermectin, and albendazole are safe drugs. They have been given to hundreds of millions of people. However, people with large numbers of microfilariae in their blood may experience fever, headache, muscle aches, and fatigue. These adverse reactions, which are caused by the death of the microfilariae, usually last no longer than 48 hours. Rest is recommended, and medicine (e.g., paracetamol) can be given for the pain and fever.

DEC also kills some of the adult worms. Adult worm death can cause a painful lump, or nodule, which begins 1–7 days after taking the drug, and may last a few weeks. In men, these painful nodules usually occur inside the scrotal sac, because this is where adult worms tend to live in men. In women, the adult worms live in the lymphatic vessels of the thigh, arm, groin, or breast, so after treatment with DEC, nodules may be found in these locations. Nodules identical to these also appear when the adult worms die "naturally", in the absence of DEC treatment.

The nodules are caused by *inflammation,* which is the body's response to the death of the adult worm. Signs of inflammation include pain, warmth, and redness. Often, the inflammation involves not only the adult worm, but also the nearby lymphatic vessel. This inflammation spreads from the site of the dead adult worm (i.e., the nodule) towards the foot or hand (i.e., away from the body, in a "retrograde" direction), causing a red, warm, tender cord just under the skin. This cord is the inflamed lymphatic vessel. The development of such a cord is known as "streaking". The medical term for an inflamed lymphatic vessel is "lymphangitis" (Fig. 1.09). Rarely, adult worm death causes lymphoedema, which resolves without treatment.

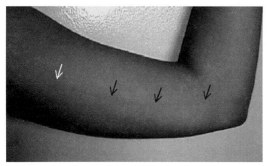

Fig. 1.09 Lymphangitis (arrows) following the death of one or more adult filarial worms. The white arrow shows the starting point of the process (the site of the dead worms). The inflammation moves along the lymphatic vessel in a retrograde direction, towards the elbow.

Even though people with these painful nodules may not feel well, they can usually continue their normal daily activities. A cool compress at the site of the nodule or along the inflamed lymphatic vessel will help relieve the pain. Rest and medicine for pain (e.g., paracetamol) are also recommended if necessary.

Unlike most individuals, pregnant women in the second or third trimester may feel very sick when adult worms die spontaneously. Any pregnant woman who has lymphangitis should be sent to the clinic for evaluation. If this is not possible, advise her to rest and to use a cold compress on the affected area. Medicine should not be given to a pregnant woman unless prescribed by a medical professional. Pregnant women should be excluded from annual mass treatment with antifilarial drugs. They can be treated safely 30 days after delivery, or during the next round of mass treatment if they are not pregnant again.

Medication for People with Microfilariae in Their Blood

In many areas where lymphatic filariasis occurs, health workers know how to take blood samples and examine the blood for microfilariae using a microscope (Fig.

1.02). People who have microfilariae in their blood should be treated with drugs to kill the worms. In some areas, these drugs may only be available during the once-a-year treatment for all members of the community. If this is the case in your area, advise anyone who is known to be microfilaria-positive about the importance of taking the antifilarial drugs during the next drug distribution.

In places without mass treatment, you should know where people can have their blood tested for microfilariae, so that you can inform your patients and other community members. If microfilariae are found in their blood, these people will need treatment with antifilarial drugs. Usually, antifilarial drugs should be available at the clinic where blood is tested for microfilariae.

If you need to know more about antifilarial drug treatment (such as drug dose, management of adverse reactions, or specific contraindications to treatment)—either for the individual patient or for mass treatment—contact the health officials in your area who are responsible for lymphatic filariasis control and elimination.

Although mass treatment with antifilarial drugs makes it possible to rid communities of filarial infection, until recently there was no hope for people who already suffered from the disease and little that could be done to help them. While there is still no *definitive* cure for those who already have lymphoedema, there are now special ways to manage the disease that are easy, inexpensive, and effective (Fig. 1.10). This is exciting news indeed, both for your patients and for you as a health care provider.

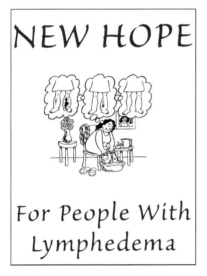

Fig. 1.10 The cover of a booklet developed for teaching patients how to care for their lymphoedema.

Thus, to achieve its goal of eliminating lymphatic filariasis as a public health problem, the Global Programme to Eliminate Lymphatic Filariasis has two major objectives. The first is to stop the spread of the filarial parasite by mosquitoes through treatment with antifilarial drugs. The second is disability prevention and rehabilitation. This book is dedicated to providing you with the information you need to prevent disability and help rehabilitate those who already suffer from the devastating long-term effects of lymphatic filariasis.

Recommended Reading

Andrade LD, Medeiros Z, Pires ML, Pimentel A, Rocha A, Figueredo-Silva J, Coutinho A, Dreyer G. Comparative efficacy of three different diethylcarbamazine regimens in lymphatic filariasis. *Trans Roy Soc Trop Med Hyg* 1995; 89:319–321.

Beach MJ, Streit TG, Addiss DG, Prospere R, Lafontant JG, Lammie PJ. Assessment of combined ivermectin and albendazole for treatment of intestinal helminth and *Wuchereria bancrofti* infections in Haitian schoolchildren. *Am J Trop Med Hyg* 1999; 60:479–486.

Dreyer G, Pires ML, Andrade LD, Lopes E, Medeiros Z, Tenorio J, Coutinho A, Noroes Figueredo-Silva J. Tolerance of diethylcarbamazine by microfilaraemic and amicrofilaraemic individuals in an endemic area of bancroftian filariasis, Recife, Brazil. *Trans Roy Soc Trop Med Hyg* 1994; 88:232–236.

Dreyer G, Medeiros A, Netto MJ, Leal NC, de Castro LG, Piessens WF. Acute attacks in the extremities of persons living in an area endemic for bancroftian filariasis: differentiation of two syndromes. *Trans Roy Soc Trop Med Hyg* 1999; 93:413–417.

Gelband H. Diethylcarbamazine salt in the control of lymphatic filariasis. *Am J Trop Med Hyg* 1994; 50:655–662.

Noroes J, Dreyer G, Santos A, Mendes VG, Medeiros Z, Addiss D. Assessment of the efficacy of diethylcarbamazine on adult *Wuchereria bancrofti in vivo. Trans Roy Soc Trop Med Hyg* 1997; 91:78–81.

Ottesen EA, Duke BOL, Karam M, Behbehani K. Strategies and tools for the control/elimination of lymphatic filariasis. *Bull World Health Org* 1997; 75:491–503.

Ottesen EA. The role of albendazole in programmes to eliminate lymphatic filariasis. *Parasitol Today* 1999;15:382–386.

Seim AR, Dreyer G, Addiss D. Controlling morbidity and interrupting transmission: twin pillars of lymphatic filariasis elimination. *Revista da Sociedade Brasileira de Medicina Tropical* 1999; 32:325–328.

World Health Organization, 1995. *World Health Report,* 1995. Geneva.

For further information on the scientific publications please contact a university or medical school library, or write to Centers for Disease Control and Prevention (contact information on page 111).

Additional copies of the Hope Club Booklet are available free of charge from Centers for Disease Control and Prevention (CDC) (contact information on page 111).

CHAPTER TWO
Filariasis and the Lymphatic Vessels

The Lymphatic System

The lymphatic system is made of lymphatic vessels (also known as lymphatics), lymph nodes, and other structures that are similar to lymph nodes, all of which are distributed throughout the body. One of the most important functions of the lymphatic system is the destruction of microscopic "intruders" such as bacteria, which can cause a variety of diseases.

Lymphatic vessels are organized as a network of tubes that move fluid and other substances from the tissues of the body back to the heart. This fluid is called lymph fluid. Thousands of tiny lymphatic vessels merge together to form larger vessels. Within these larger vessels, lymph fluid can move in one direction only, towards the heart (Fig. 2.01).

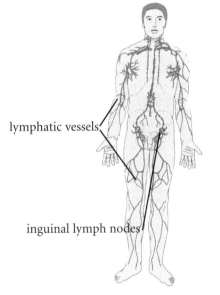

lymphatic vessels

inguinal lymph nodes

Fig. 2.01 The lymphatic system (shown in blue) is made of a network of lymphatic vessels and lymph nodes.

The main function of the lymphatic vessels is to remove waste material from the tissues of the body. This process also removes excess water and sends a variety of infectious organisms, such as bacteria, to the lymph nodes, where they are destroyed.

Exercise helps remove excess water from the tissues. When muscles tighten around a lymphatic vessel, they push the fluid inside the vessel towards the heart.

The reduced capacity of lymphatics to remove these substances from the tissues and transport them to the heart is known as *lymphatic insufficiency*. Anything that damages the lymphatic vessels can cause lymphatic insufficiency. Two examples include birth defects (which result in a decreased number of healthy lymphatic vessels), and the adult worms of lymphatic filariasis. Insufficiency of the lymphatics leads to lymphatic dysfunction, which, alone or in combination with other factors, can cause lymphoedema.

Many small lymphatic vessels are located in the skin, including the skin of the feet, penis, and scrotum. Bacteria can be found in large numbers on the surface of the skin, especially in these areas. From time to time they reach the lymphatic system but are usually destroyed without causing any sign of infection.

Lymph nodes are found at certain points along the lymphatic vessels (Fig. 2.01). The lymph nodes filter bacteria from the lymph fluid. When the lymph nodes trap large numbers of bacteria they grow large and tender. They feel like lumps underneath the skin.

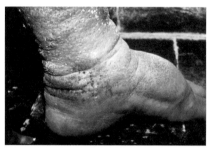

Fig. 2.02 Lymphoedema and dirty skin. Many bacteria can be found on the skin when patients do not wash properly.

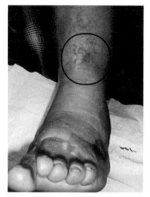

Fig. 2.03 A break in the skin (circle). Because bacteria can enter the skin at this point and cause an acute attack, breaks in the skin are called "entry lesions."

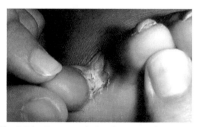

Fig. 2.04 An entry lesion between the toes—a very common site for entry lesions.

Adult Filarial Worms Damage the Lymphatic Vessels

When adult filarial worms live in lymphatic vessels, they cause the vessels to dilate, or become larger. This process, known as dilatation, disturbs the function of the lymphatic vessels, and can change the flow of lymph fluid, leading to lymphatic insufficiency. Thus, when adult worms dilate the lymphatic vessels, the vessels do not work properly.

The location of the lymphatic vessel damage influences the type of disease that your patient will develop. When the damaged lymphatic vessels drain the skin, the patient is at risk of developing lymphoedema. When damaged lymphatic vessels drain deeper tissues, such as the testicles or the urinary tract, other clinical manifestations may occur.

Consequences of Damaged Lymphatic Vessels Draining the Skin

Patients with damaged lymphatic vessels and lymphoedema often have more bacteria on the skin than usual (Fig. 2.02) because they are unable or do not know how to wash properly. They also usually have small cuts, breaks, or scratches in the skin (Fig. 2.03) and between the toes (Fig. 2.04), called entry lesions. Entry lesions allow large numbers of bacteria to enter the skin, and the bacteria multiply quickly. The lymph nodes are not able to filter such large numbers of bacteria. Large numbers of bacteria under the skin

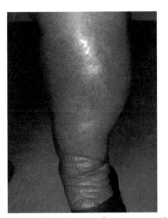

Fig. 2.05 The early stage of an acute attack. The skin is inflamed: swollen, red, hot, and very painful. The skin is also shiny, a sign that this patient has early-stage lymphoedema.

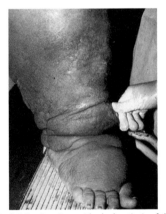

Fig. 2.06 A patient with elephantiasis of the leg. After repeated acute attacks the skin becomes harder and thicker.

cause the inflammation that is characteristic of an acute attack (Fig. 2.05). This inflammation damages the tiny lymphatic vessels in the skin, and reduces their ability to drain lymph fluid. The result is lymphoedema. After a few acute attacks, the skin becomes swollen and begins to get hard. Repeated acute attacks cause the leg, arm, breast, penis, or scrotum to increase in volume and the skin to become harder (Fig. 2.06). A "vicious cycle" begins: as the chronic swelling of the skin increases, the risk of repeated bacterial infection increases too.

Usually in lymphatic filariasis, lymphoedema appears in only one part of the body, but bilateral disease (on both sides) can occur in the legs. If a patient has generalized swelling (for example, of the legs, arms, abdomen, and face), other diseases, such as heart failure or kidney problems, are much more likely the cause of the swelling.

Lymphatic vessel damage caused by the adult filarial worm does not, in itself, produce lymphoedema. "Filarial" lymphoedema first appears after one or more (often several) acute attacks caused by bacterial infections of the skin. Patients whose swelling begins without any pain or inflammation are likely to have underlying diseases other than lymphatic filariasis, and should be referred to a clinic for further evaluation. Prompt referral at the first sign of such swelling is especially important for children and adolescents (see chapter 8).

The major goal of lymphoedema management in filariasis-endemic areas is to prevent acute attacks caused by bacterial infections. For people with no signs of lymphoedema, but whose lymphatic vessels are already damaged by filarial worms, preventing the initial acute attack will avoid the appearance of lymphoedema. For patients with lymphoedema, preventing recurrent acute attacks will halt the progressive course of lymphoedema and elephantiasis.

As we shall see in chapter 4, hygiene (Fig. 2.07) and treatment of entry lesions are extremely important measures for managing lymphoedema. Hygiene reduces the number of bacteria on the skin, and treatment of entry lesions reduces the ability of bacteria to enter the skin.

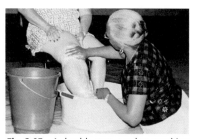

Fig. 2.07 A health care worker teaching good hygiene to a patient with lymphoedema of the leg.

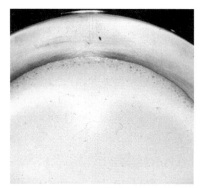

Fig. 2.08 Milky-white urine from a patient with chyluria.

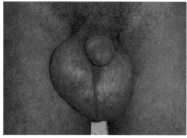

Fig. 2.09 The genitals of a man with hydrocoele. The volume of the scrotal sac is larger than normal on both sides. The penis is normal.

Consequences of Damaged Lymphatic Vessels Draining Sites Other Than the Skin

If the adult filarial worms live in other lymphatic vessels that are *not* directly linked to the skin, the patient may develop other forms of filarial disease, such as milky urine—known as chyluria—(Fig. 2.08), and excess fluid inside the scrotal sac—known as hydrocoele (Fig. 2.09). These conditions are discussed further in Chapter 6.

Filariasis and the Lymphatic System in Children

In children, lymphatic filariasis does not cause the chronic forms of swelling described above, such as lymphoedema and hydrocoele. However, adult filarial worms can be found in children, even in those less than 5 years old. In children, the adult worms affect primarily the lymph nodes, causing the nodes to become large (Fig. 2.10) and, occasionally, painful. As a health worker, you know that other diseases also affect the lymph nodes in children. Children with enlarged lymph nodes, especially if there are several nodes or they are very large, should be referred to a clinic for further evaluation.

As children get older, especially during the early teenage years, the preferential site of the living adult worms of *Wuchereria bancrofti* becomes the lymphatic vessels, as described above for the adult population.

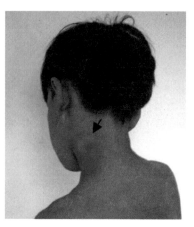

Fig. 2.10 Lymph node (arrow). In children, enlarged lymph nodes are very common. In addition to many other diseases, an enlarged lymph node may be a sign of lymphatic filariasis. Enlarged lymph nodes, which affect boys and girls equally, can appear anywhere on the body.

Recommended Reading

Amaral F, Dreyer G, Figueredo-Silva J, Norões J, Cavalcanti A, Samico SF, Santo A, Coutinho A. Live adult worms detected by ultrasonography in human bancroftian filariasis. *Am J Trop Med Hyg* 1994; 50:753–757.

Dreyer G, Norões J, Addiss D, Santos A, Medeiros Z, Figueredo-Silva J. Bancroftian filariasis in a pediatric population: An ultrasonographic study. *Trans Roy Soc Trop Med Hyg* 1999; 93:633–636.

Dreyer G, Norões J, Figueredo-Silva J. Elimination of lymphatic filariasis as a public health problem. New insights into the natural history and pathology of bancroftian filariasis: implications for clinical management and filariasis control programs. *Trans Roy Soc Trop Med Hyg* 2000; 94:594–596.

Dreyer G, Norões J, Figueredo-Silva J, Piessens WF. Pathogenesis of lymphatic disease in bancroftian filariasis: A clinical perspective. *Parasitol Today* 2000; 16:544–548.

Dreyer G, Addiss D, Roberts J, Norões J. Progression of lymphatic vessel dilatation in the presence of living adult *Wuchereria bancrofti*. *Trans Roy Soc Trop Med Hyg,* in press.

Dreyer G, Figueredo-Silva J, Carvalho K, Amaral F, Ottesen EA. Lymphatic filariasis in children: adenopathy and its evolution in two young girls. *Am J Trop Med Hyg,* 2001; 65:204–207.

Figueredo-Silva J, Dreyer G, Guimaraes K, Brandt C, Medeiros Z. Bancroftian lymphadenopathy: absence of eosinophils in tissues despite peripheral blood hypereosinophilia. *J Trop Med Hyg* 1994; 97:55–59.

Jungmann P, Figueredo-Silva J, Dreyer G. Bancroftian lymphadenopathy: a histopathologic study of fifty-eight cases from Northeastern Brazil. *Am J Trop Med Hyg* 1991; 45:325–331.

Jungmann P, Figueredo-Silva J, Dreyer G. Bancroftian lymphangitis in Northeastern Brazil: a histopathological study of 17 cases. *J Trop Med Hyg* 1992; 95:114–118.

Lammie PJ, Reiss MD, Dimock KA, Streit TG, Roberts JM, Eberhard, ML. Longitudinal analysis of the development of filarial infection and antifilarial immunity in a cohort of Haitian children. *Am J Trop Med Hyg* 1998; 59:217–221.

Marchetti F, Piessens FW, Medeiros Z, Dreyer G. Abnormalities in the leg lymphatics are not specific for bancroftian filariasis. *Trans Roy Soc Trop Med Hyg* 1998; 92:650–652.

Norões J, Addiss D, Santos A, Medeiros Z, Coutinho A, Dreyer G. Ultrasonographic evidence of abnormal lymphatic vessels in young men with adult *Wuchereria bancrofti* infection in the scrotal area. *J Urol* 1996; 156: 409–412.

Olszewski WL, Jamal S, Dworozynski A, Swoboda E, Pani SP, Manokaran GVK, Bryla P. Bacteriological studies of skin, tissue fluid and lymph in filarial lymphoedema. *Lymphology* 1994; 27(Suppl):345–348.

Shenoy RK, Sandha K, Suma TK, Kumaraswami V. A preliminary study of filariasis related to acute lymphangitis with special reference to precipitating factors and treatment modalities. *Southeast Asian J Trop Med Pub Health* 1995; 26:301–305.

Shenoy RK, Suma TK, Rajan K, Kumaraswami V. Prevention of acute lymphangitis in brugian filariasis: comparison of the efficacy of ivermectin and diethylcarbamazine, each combined with local treatment of the affected limb. *Ann Trop Med Parasitol* 1998; 92:587–594.

Witt C, Ottesen EA. Lymphatic filariasis: An infection in childhood. *Trop Med Internat Health* 2001; 6:582–606.

For further information on the scientific publications please contact a university or medical school library, or write to Centers for Disease Control and Prevention (contact information on page 111).

CHAPTER THREE
Assessment of Chronic Lymphoedema

Being able to determine the stage of lymphoedema will allow you to choose the proper management and to advise your patients on how their disease may progress. Lymphoedema staging is also useful at the community level. If program managers know the number of patients in a given area and the stage of their lymphoedema, they can more effectively develop plans and budgets for programs to care for these patients.

The following classification for lymphoedema of lymphatic filariasis uses 7 stages. Stage 1 represents early or mild disease, while stage 7 is the most severe. The stages do not describe the natural history of lymphoedema at the individual level, and they are not necessarily progressive. For example, patients with stage 6 lymphoedema may never have had the features characteristic of stage 4 or 5 lymphoedema. However, lymphoedema stages are related to severity of disease, to the risk of acute attacks, and to the complexity and intensity of lymphoedema management.

Features Used for Staging

- *Is the swelling reversible overnight?*
  (reversible swelling: disappears spontaneously overnight)
- *Are there any shallow skin folds?*
  (shallow fold: the base of the fold is visible when the patient moves the leg or foot so that the fold "opens up")
- *Are knobs present?*
  (knobs: bumps, lumps, or protrusions of the skin)
- *Are there any deep skin folds?*
  (deep fold: the base is visible only when the edges of the fold are separated by hand)
- *Are mossy lesions present?*
  (mossy lesions: clusters of small growths on the skin, usually on the foot, with a peculiar wart-like appearance)
- *Is the patient unable to adequately or independently perform routine daily activities?*

In addition to using these features, each lymphoedema patient should be assessed for the following conditions:

- entry lesions in the skin folds (Fig. 3.01) and between the toes (Fig. 3.02) and fingers (Fig. 3.03)

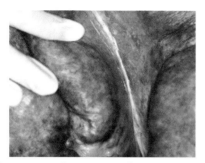

Fig. 3.01 Entry lesion in a deep fold in a patient with elephantiasis of the leg.

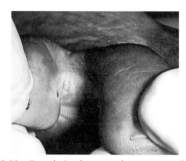

Fig. 3.02 Entry lesion between the toes, caused by a fungal infection. Entry lesions that lead to repeated acute attacks are most commonly found between the toes.

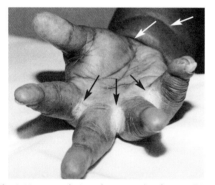

Fig. 3.03 Entry lesions between the fingers (black arrows) in a patient with stage 3 lymphoedema of the arm. Note the skin folds (white arrow), which are shallow (the base of the fold is visible when the patient moves the wrist). Note also the similarity of these entry lesions with those found between the toes (Fig. 3.02).

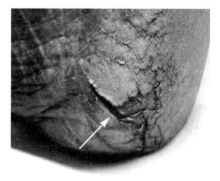

Fig. 3.04 Cracks in the sole of the foot. Patients with lymphoedema commonly have cracks in the soles of the feet (arrow), especially if they walk barefoot.

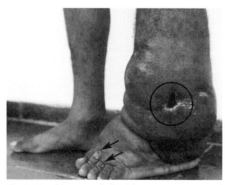

Fig. 3.05 Skin wound (circle) in a patient with lymphoedema of the leg. Two isolated knobs at the base of the toes are indicated by arrows.

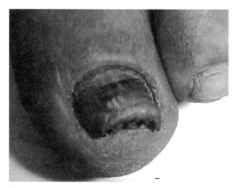

Fig. 3.06 Onychomycosis, or fungal infection of the nails. Fungal infection of the nails is very common in many parts of the world, not only in filariasis-endemic areas.

- bad odour
- cracks in the sole of the foot (Fig. 3.04)
- wounds of any kind on the surface of the leg or foot (Fig. 3.05)
- fungal infections of the nails (onychomycosis) (Fig 3.06)
- venous insufficiency (see chapter 7)

Although these conditions are not used for staging, they are used, along with the frequency of acute attacks, to monitor patient progress. The size of the leg, or leg volume, tends to increase with higher stages, but patients can have severe disease and still have a leg that is almost normal in size.

This classification applies to lymphoedema of the arms or legs. Because the legs are the most common sites of lymphoedema in filariasis-endemic areas, we will refer primarily to the leg in this book. Lymphoedema also occurs in the breast, penis, and scrotum, but the stages presented here for the arms and legs do not apply to lymphoedema elsewhere. However, the basic principles of treatment are the same.

The following tips will help you to stage lymphoedema correctly:

- Stage the right side and left side separately. They often are not the same stage.
- On each side, stage the foot and the leg together.
- If signs of more than one stage exist, the leg and foot are classified by the higher stage. For example, if the leg has shallow skin folds (Stage 3) and there are mossy lesions on the foot (Stage 6), the leg will be classified as Stage 6.
- During an acute attack, it may not be possible to accurately stage lymphoedema in early stages. Ideally, the lymphoedema should be staged only after recovery (usually 30 days after an acute attack).
- Stages can change with treatment. To document improvement in stage of lymphoedema, the patient should be classified before treatment begins.

Special reminder: Don't forget that patients can have entry lesions and lymphoedema in more than one place. When assessing the patient for lymphoedema of the leg, examine the healthy leg, the upper limbs and breasts for entry lesions and early lymphoedema, even if the patient doesn't have any other complaints.

Stage 1

The feature of stage 1 lymphoedema is:

- Swelling is reversible (goes away) overnight.

In stage 1 lymphoedema, the swelling increases during the day and goes away overnight when the patient lies flat in bed, not because of any specific treatment (Fig. 3.07). To accurately classify lymphoedema in patients with stage 1 disease, it is preferable to examine the leg in the late afternoon, when the swelling is most visible, and again early in the morning, to see that the swelling is gone. For patients with stage 1 lymphoedema in both legs, it is necessary to rely on the patient's report of normal-size legs in the morning, because direct comparison is more difficult.

A patient with stage 1 lymphoedema rarely has acute attacks, entry lesions, or a bad odour.

Stage 1 lymphoedema can be particularly useful from an epidemiologic perspective for assessing the prevalence of lymphoedema in young people and for monitoring the incidence of new cases of lymphoedema in communities with lymphoedema treatment programs.

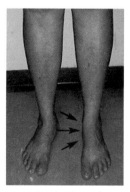

FIG. 3.07 Stage 1 lymphoedema. If you look carefully you will notice that the left leg is slightly swollen (arrows).

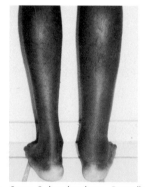

Fig. 3.08 Stage 2 lymphoedema. Regardless of the time of day, the swelling in stage 2 lymphoedema is obvious, especially if it is compared to the other leg, if that leg is normal.

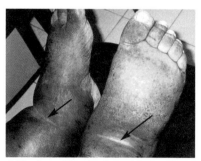

Fig. 3.09 Stage 3 lymphoedema of the leg. The arrows show the base of the shallow skin folds at the ankles.

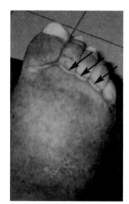

Fig. 3.10 Stage 3 lymphoedema of the toes and foot. When the patient moves the toes, the base of the shallow folds is visible (arrows). Compare with figure 3.09. Remember to look for folds at the base of the toes.

Stage 2

The feature of stage 2 lymphoedema is:

- Swelling is not reversible (does not go away) overnight.

The main difference between stage 2 lymphoedema (Fig. 3.08) and stage 1 is that the swelling does not go away without lymphoedema management. Occasionally, patients with stage 2 lymphoedema will have acute attacks. They may have entry lesions, or mild bad odour.

Stage 3

The feature of stage 3 lymphoedema is:

- Shallow skin folds.

The principal feature of stage 3 lymphoedema is the presence of one or more shallow skin folds (Figs. 3.09 and 3.10). Shallow folds are those in which the base of the fold can be seen when the patient moves the leg or foot so that the fold "opens up". Even very thin lines or creases, which are not seen on normal legs, are considered shallow folds. Early shallow folds are much easier to see when the patient is standing. Thus, it is important to have the patient standing when you are staging the lymphoedema.

Patients with stage 3 lymphoedema may have occasional acute attacks. Entry lesions between the toes and bad odour are more common than in stage 2.

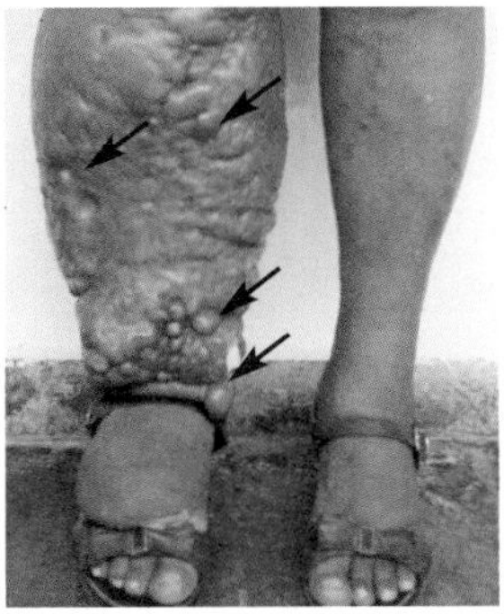

Stage 4

The feature of stage 4 lymphoedema is:

- Knobs.

Fig. 3.11 Stage 4 lymphoedema. This patient has multiple knobs (arrows).

Knobs are bumps, lumps, or protrusions of the skin (Fig. 3.11). The importance of knobs as a feature of stage 4 lymphoedema comes from fact that knobs predispose the leg to further trauma and, therefore, to additional entry lesions, especially if the skin at the site of the knob is less sensitive than the surrounding skin.

In some filariasis-endemic areas, people may be prone to develop protruding scars known as keloids. These scars are also classified as knobs (Fig. 3.12) because they represent an abnormal healing process at the site of an earlier entry lesion, and because the patient may be predisposed to further trauma at this site, where the sensitivity of skin is reduced.

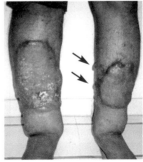

Fig. 3.12 Stage 4 lymphoedema. Large knobs produced by scars on both legs. Note two small protruding knobs on the inside of the left leg (arrows). The knob on the right leg has multiple entry lesions.

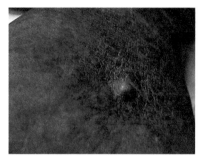

Fig. 3.13 Varicose button. Because it protrudes and is prone to trauma, this dilated vein should be classified as a knob (see chapter 7).

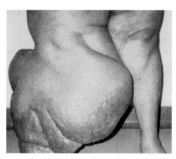

Fig. 3.14 Stage 5 lymphoedema. This patient has multiple deep folds and large leg volume.

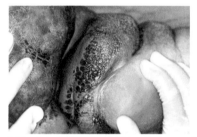

Fig. 3.15 Deep fold and very dirty skin in a patient with stage 5 lymphoedema. The base of a deep fold can be seen only when the edges of the fold are actively separated by hand.

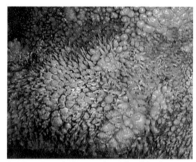

Fig. 3.16 Mossy lesion on the side of the foot, near the heel. Note that some of these structures are elongated, or fusiform, while others are rounded.

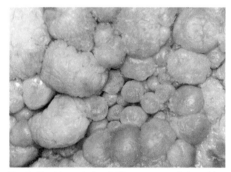

Fig. 3.17 Mossy lesion with many rounded vesicles, shown at high magnification. The vesicles are very delicate and they rupture as a result of minor trauma. Special care must be taken to avoid rupturing the vesicles during the process of washing and drying.

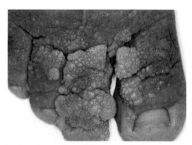

Fig. 3.18 Mossy foot. This is a typical mossy wart-like lesion in a patient with stage 6 lymphoedema.

As will be discussed in Chapter 7, patients who not only have lymphoedema and lymphatic insufficiency, but also *venous insufficiency,* may have dilated, twisted veins that lie very close to the surface of the skin. In some places, these veins protrude, creating what is called a "varicose button" (Fig. 3.13). Varicose buttons should be considered as knobs, even if the rest of the skin is smooth. Varicose buttons are prone to trauma and can serve as potential entry lesions.

Patients with stage 4 lymphoedema experience occasional acute attacks. Many patients will have entry lesions between the toes and a bad odour.

Stage 5

The feature of stage 5 lymphoedema is:

• Deep skin folds.

The presence of one or more deep skin folds is the main feature of stage 5 lymphoedema (Fig. 3.14). Deep folds are those whose base cannot be seen when the patient moves the leg or foot so that the fold "opens up"; rather, the base of the fold can be seen only when the edges are actively separated by hand (Fig. 3.15).

Patients with stage 5 lymphoedema experience occasional to frequent acute attacks. Most patients will have entry lesions between the toes or in the folds, as well as a bad odour.

Stage 6

The feature of stage 6 lymphoedema is:

• Mossy lesions.

On the surface of the skin (especially the upper surface of the toes), small elongated (Fig. 3.16) or rounded growths (Fig. 3.17) are clustered together, giving rise to the peculiar appearance of "mossy lesions". When located on the foot, this condition is known as "mossy foot" (Fig. 3.18). Rarely, these lesions can appear on the leg (Figs. 3.19 and 3.20).

It may not be easy to distinguish between very small knobs and early mossy lesions (Fig 3.21). If you are in doubt, it may be helpful to shine a bright light on the lesion (Fig. 3.22). Mossy lesions contain fluid (Fig. 3.17), and are transparent or translucent (light can shine through them). In contrast, knobs do not allow light to pass through. Mossy lesions usually leak fluid, which puts the patient at high risk of bacterial infection.

Patients with stage 6 lymphoedema have acute attacks. Almost all patients with stage 6 lymphoedema have entry lesions between the toes and a bad odour. The toenails may be destroyed (Fig 3.23). Wounds in the skin frequently are present.

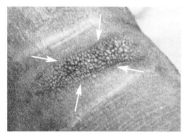

Fig. 3.19 Early mossy lesion (arrows) between shallow folds where the foot meets the leg. This is an unusual location for a mossy lesion. It is necessary to distinguish early mossy lesions from small knobs (see Fig. 3.21).

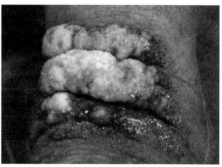

Fig. 3.20 Advanced mossy lesion, with wart-like growths, on the lower leg just above the foot.

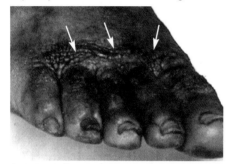

Fig. 3.21 Early mossy lesion. Even though it is unusual for knobs to appear in clusters near the toes (arrows), it is important to differentiate these mossy lesions (stage 6 lymphoedema) from knobs (stage 4 lymphoedema), because the management of the patient and the prognosis are different.

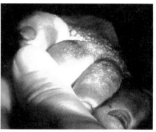

Fig. 3.22 Knobs or mossy lesions? A light can help you differentiate between knobs (light does not pass through them) and mossy lesions (light passes through the vesicles—they are translucent).

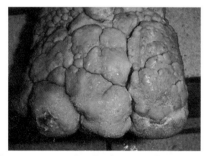

Fig. 3.23 Stage 6 lymphoedema. In advanced mossy foot, the nails are destroyed. Some pieces of the nails may remain loosely attached. During hygiene it is important not to try to remove them forcefully. Nails that are already destroyed but are still attached to the toes will detach spontaneously in time.

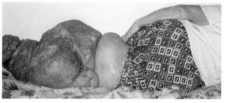

Fig. 3.24 Stage 7 lymphoedema. This patient's leg has a very large volume and many entry lesions. This patient is disabled and requires help for her daily activities.

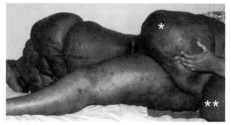

Fig. 3.25 Stage 7 lymphoedema. This patient has elephantiasis of the leg and lymphoedema of the abdomen (*) and breast (**). Lymphoedema of the abdomen and breast are not staged by this classification system.

Stage 7

The feature of stage 7 lymphoedema is:

- The patient is unable to adequately or independently perform routine daily activities such as walking, bathing, or cooking, etc.

Patients with stage 7 lymphoedema (Figs. 3.24 and 3.25) have frequent acute attacks and large legs, usually with deep folds. They always have entry lesions between the toes and skin folds. The bad odour is very strong. Wounds in the skin are commonly present, and lymphoedema extends above the knee in most patients.

The principal feature of stage 7 lymphoedema is that the patient cannot perform daily activities. Assistance from the family and the health care system is needed.

> **Warning:** *If patients with stage 7 lymphoedema have been confined to bed for a long time, do not attempt to move or ask them to walk without medical supervision. They can break a bone, especially in the diseased leg, or they may even die suddenly as a result of a blood clot in the leg going to the lung (pulmonary embolism).*

The following table summarizes the features for each stage of lymphoedema.

OVERVIEW OF FEATURES USED TO STAGE LYMPHOEDEMA

Feature	Stage 1	Stage 2	Stage 3	Stage 4	Stage 5	Stage 6	Stage 7
Leg swelling	Goes away without treatment	Permanent, without treatment	Permanent	Permanent	Permanent; may extend above the knee	Permanent; may be mild or severe	Permanent; usually extends above the knee
Skin folds	Absent	Absent	Shallow	Shallow folds can be present	Deep. With or without shallow folds	Any type of fold can be present	Any type of fold can be present
Knobs	Absent	Absent	Absent	Present	Present or Absent	Present or Absent	Present or Absent
Mossy lesions	Absent	Absent	Absent	Absent	Absent	Present	Present or Absent
Severely disabled	No	No	No	No	No	No	Yes

Recommended Viewing

Lymphatic Filariasis: Hope for a better life. (Training video). Program for patients, 21 minutes. Program for health care workers, 58 minutes.

Copies of the video may be purchased through the Public Health Foundation in the United States (contact information on page 111).

CHAPTER FOUR
Lymphoedema Management

The Need for Lymphoedema Management

The damage that adult filarial worms cause to the lymphatic system is permanent. Antifilarial drugs will not cure lymphoedema. However, lymphoedema can be managed by stopping acute attacks and preventing the disease from getting worse.

If lymphoedema is not managed properly and the disease progresses, patients will find it more difficult to work or go to school. They frequently will feel alone and may lose their friends, family, and jobs. Good lymphoedema management can give your patients new hope for a better life.

Lymphoedema management also gives other benefits:

- It eliminates the bad odour.
- It prevents and heals entry lesions.
- It improves patients' self-confidence.
- It often reduces the size of the leg, arm, or other affected area.
- It improves patients' ability to work or go to school.

The Basic Components of Lymphoedema Management

The management of lymphoedema has five components: hygiene (Fig. 4.01), prevention and cure of entry lesions (Fig. 4.02), exercise (Fig. 4.03), elevation (Fig. 4.04) and wearing proper shoes (Fig. 4.05).

How do these components work?

Hygiene and care of entry lesions prevent acute attacks. Washing removes most of the bacteria from the skin surface (Fig. 4.06, 4.07). Cure and prevention of entry lesions keep these bacteria from entering the skin. If entry lesions exist between the toes and folds, or if there are wounds (such as cuts, scratches, or cracks) on the skin, bacteria are able to enter the skin and cause infection. This can lead to an acute attack (Fig. 4.08).

Reducing the extra fluid in the leg also helps to prevent bacterial infections. Exercise and elevation help move fluid from the affected limb back to the heart. Shoes protect the feet from trauma and entry lesions. Patients can add these simple measures to their daily activities.

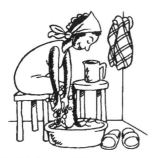

Fig. 4.01 Daily hygiene will prevent the acute attacks and it takes only a little of your patient's time.

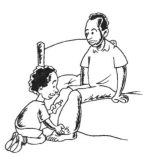

Fig. 4.02 After washing and drying the legs, the helper is applying medicated cream to heal the entry lesions.

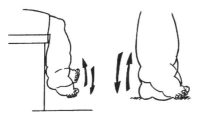

Fig. 4.03 Exercise can be done everywhere, and it does not cost anything.

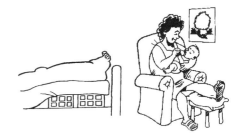

Fig. 4.04 The leg can be elevated frequently, for example, while the patient rests or feeds the baby.

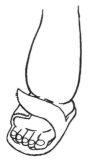

Fig. 4.05 Comfortable shoes are an important component of lymphoedema management.

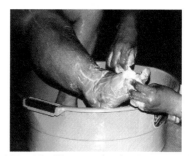

Fig. 4.06 A health care worker showing a patient how to remove most of the bacteria from the skin, paying special attention to the area between the toes.

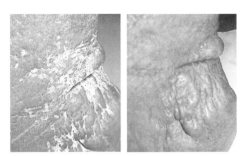

Fig. 4.07 An example of the results of good hygiene. On the left, the patient's leg before washing; on the right, after a few days of daily washing. The bad odour completely disappeared.

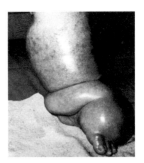

Fig. 4.08 A patient with a severe acute attack of the leg. Note the shiny swollen skin, which is very painful.

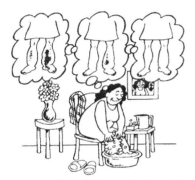

Fig. 4.09 Hope. The patient knows that by washing her legs every day, she will improve the condition of her lymphoedema. Share this message with your patients.

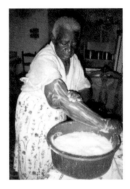

Fig. 4.10 Washing the arm. The patient is standing to demonstrate how well she can do the washing herself.

Steps in Lymphoedema Management

The following pages explain the steps of lymphoedema management. At the end of the chapter, these steps are organized into a management plan for each of the seven different stages of lymphoedema. Patients who follow the steps of lymphoedema management will notice an improvement in their condition (Fig. 4.09).

STEP 1. HYGIENE – WASHING

Although the following steps refer to the leg, hygiene should also be used for lymphoedema of the arm (Fig. 4.10), breast, and genital area (see chapter 6). In addition, even if a patient has lymphoedema in only one leg, both legs must be washed.

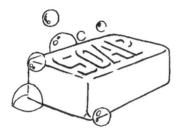

Fig. 4.11 Soap. The least expensive soap without perfume is usually suitable for your patients.

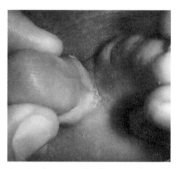

Fig. 4.12 Another example of an entry lesion between the toes. This one can be seen only if one looks carefully, but it still can allow bacteria to enter, causing an acute attack. It will be cured just by washing and carefully drying.

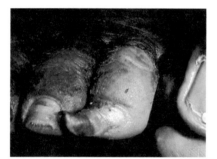

Fig. 4.13 Long toenails. Many patients need help with trimming their nails, especially those with advanced lymphoedema. This must be done carefully to avoid creating additional entry lesions.

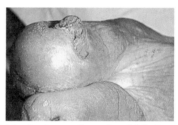

Fig. 4.14 Onychomycosis, or fungal infection of the nail. Uncomplicated onychomycosis itself does not predispose to acute bacterial infections. Cleaning under the nail should only be done after washing, and when advised by a health worker. Patients should be discouraged from attempting to clean under the nail with sharp objects, which can cut the skin and create entry lesions.

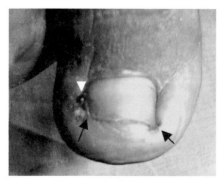

Fig. 4.15 Ingrown toenail. The patient trimmed his toenails incorrectly, and the growing edges of the nail are digging into the toe (black arrows). A small entry lesion can already be seen (white arrow).

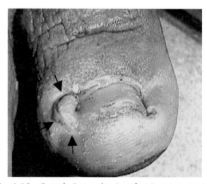

Fig. 4.16 Entry lesion at the site of an ingrown toenail, same patient as in Fig. 4.15, seven days later. The lesion has been washed well in preparation for surgically removing the abnormal tissue (arrows). Ingrown toenails can be dangerous entry lesions for your patients.

1.1. Prepare a place to wash the legs. The supplies needed are:

- *clean* water at room temperature
- soap (Fig. 4.11)
- a basin
- a chair or stool
- a towel
- and shoes. Put the shoes within easy reach.

1.2. Always start by checking the skin for:

- Entry lesions, including very small lesions between the toes that hardly can be seen (Fig. 4.12). It is important to check the skin every time the leg is washed because entry lesions allow bacteria to enter, and this will cause acute attacks. If entry lesions are found, they should be cleaned carefully.
- Toenails that need trimming (Fig. 4.13). Always trim the toenails after washing, when they are softer. Patients with extensive fungal infection of the toenails (onychomycosis) may prefer to have a few nails trimmed each day for several days in a row, rather than all at once. In patients who have fungal infections of the nails (Fig. 4.14), do not try to clean under the nails with sharp objects. If your patient has an ingrown toenail that is causing problems (Figs. 4.15 and 4.16), refer her or him to someone who is trained to treat this condition. Ingrown toenails are more dangerous than many other entry lesions as triggers of an acute attack. Patients with lymphoedema are free to use nail polish (Fig. 4.17), but advise them not to remove the cuticles (Fig. 4.18).

1.3. Wash the affected leg

- Before washing the leg, wash the hands.
- Wet the leg with clean water at room temperature.
- Lather the hands with the soap, rather than putting soap directly on the leg.
- Begin soaping at the highest point of swelling (usually around the knee) (Fig. 4.19).
- Wash down the leg towards the foot.
- Gently clean between all skin folds and between the toes. A small cloth (Fig. 4.20) or cotton swab will make this more effective. Pay particular attention to entry lesions.
- Brushes should not be used, as they can damage the skin.
- Rinse with clean water.
- Repeat this careful washing until the rinse water is no longer dirty.
- Wash the other leg in the same way, even if it looks normal.

> *Reminder: Hot or warm water should not be used to wash the leg that has lymphoedema. Use water that is at room temperature or cooler.*

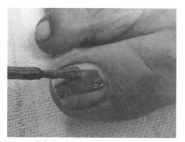

Fig. 4.17 Polishing the nails. This is not a harmful practice for the patient with lymphoedema. If polishing the nails is acceptable in your culture as a sign of adornment or beauty, you can even encourage your patients to do so.

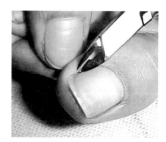

Fig. 4.18 Removal of the cuticle—a harmful practice. Removing the cuticle can create entry lesions and put your patient at risk of acute attacks. Tell your patients with lymphoedema *not* to cut or try to remove the cuticles.

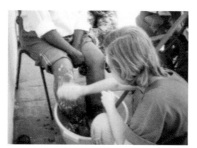

Fig. 4.19 The health care worker instructs the patient to wash the leg in a downward direction: from the knee towards the foot.

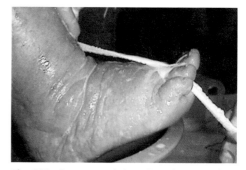

Fig. 4.20 Use a soapy cloth or piece of gauze to clean between the toes.

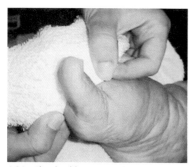

Fig. 4.21 The health care worker is showing the patient how to dry between the toes after washing.

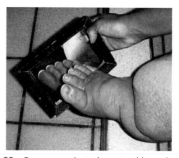

Fig. 4.22 Do your patients have trouble seeing their entry lesions? You can show them how to make this search easier by using a mirror.

1.4. Dry the skin well

- Pat the area lightly with a clean towel. Do not rub hard because this can damage the skin.
- Carefully dry (Fig 4.21) between the toes and between skin folds using a small towel, cloth, gauze, or cotton swab.
- For some patients, such as those with mossy lesions, drying may be difficult. In these cases, after drying with a towel, air-drying with a fan (either hand-held or electric) is recommended.

STEP 2. MANAGEMENT OF ENTRY LESIONS AFTER HYGIENE

Entry lesions are particularly common in patients with lymphoedema. They are most frequently found where it is warm and moist: between the toes, in the deep skin folds, and around the toenails. Entry lesions, such as wounds, can also be found on the surface of the skin. A mirror can be used to examine for entry lesions in places that are difficult to see (Fig. 4.22).

Both fungi and bacteria can cause entry lesions. Fungal infections frequently damage the skin and create entry lesions, especially between the toes and in skin folds (Fig 4.23). These entry lesions allow bacteria to enter the body through the skin, and this can cause acute attacks. Fungi and bacteria can cause a bad odour. This odour is especially offensive when it is caused by bacteria that live in deep folds; these bacteria are anaerobic—they do not require air to grow.

After washing, look again carefully between the toes and in the shallow and deep skin folds for entry lesions. Between the toes, the colour of fungal infections is usually white (Fig. 4.24) or pink (Fig. 4.25). Fungal infections usually do not leak fluid. In contrast, bacterial infections may leak fluid that is thin and clear, or thick and yellow (Fig. 4.26), green, or brownish in colour.

A variety of antiseptics and antifungal and antibacterial agents are effective in treating entry lesions that do not heal with hygiene alone. Their availability and cost vary in different regions.

2.1. Antiseptics

Antiseptics are used when antibiotic cream is not available or is too costly. They are particularly useful for patients with advanced lymphoedema because systemic antibiotics may not reach all parts of a wound in these patients. In addition, antiseptics are used in deep folds, where bacteria grow easily to large numbers and where entry lesions occur frequently.

The doctor or medical officer in charge of the lymphoedema treatment programme in your country can recommend the most suitable antiseptic for your patients in terms of availability, cost, effectiveness, and safety. Examples of antiseptics that may be recommended include potassium permanganate, hypochlorite solutions, acetic acid, povidone iodine, and cetrimide.

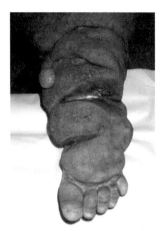

Fig. 4.23 Fungal infection, white in colour, in a shallow fold. The patient also has deep folds and a knob. Her lymphoedema will be classified as stage 5.

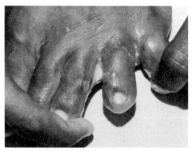

Fig. 4.24 Fungal infections, white in colour, are very common between the toes.

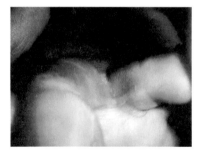

Fig. 4.25 A pink entry lesion is shown here. Teach your patient how to identify entry lesions between the toes.

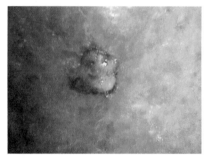

Fig. 4.26 A skin wound that is infected with bacteria. Note the yellow secretion known as pus.

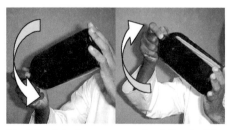

Fig. 4.27 Potassium permanganate solution should be shaken well and stored in a dark container.

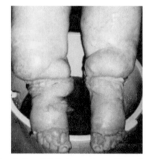

Fig. 4.28 Cotton fabric is soaked with potassium permanganate solution and placed between the folds and toes.

Even when used properly, some antiseptics can cause irritation of the skin. Patients whose entry lesions worsen or do not improve with antiseptics should stop using them and be referred to a clinic for further evaluation. For patients who respond well, the antiseptics can be discontinued after improvement is observed.

In this book, antiseptics are recommended for cleansing and disinfecting entry lesions, not for debriding wounds (removing dead tissue from the wounds). If wounds require debriding, this should be done under appropriate supervision in a clinic.

Potassium permanganate is widely used in lymphoedema programs in Brazil and Haiti and has been shown to be safe when used properly.

How to use potassium permanganate:
- The potassium permanganate solution preferably should be made fresh every day by adding a tablet or powder to clean water and shaking well (Fig. 4.27). Use one-half to 1 litre of the permanganate solution for each leg. The correct concentration is 100 milligrams of potassium permanganate for each litre of water. The tablets or powder and the solution should be stored in a dark container, because sunlight reduces the strength of potassium permanganate.
- Place the leg in a tub or basin.
- Soak any thin, clean, cotton cloth or gauze with the solution. Place pieces of the gauze or cloth inside the deep skin folds and between the toes (Fig. 4.28). If there are wounds on the skin surface, loosely wrap the cloth around the leg.
- Pour the potassium permanganate over the cloth-covered leg (Fig 4.29). As the solution collects in the basin, pour it back over the leg.
- Leave the potassium permanganate on the skin a few minutes (5–10 minutes). Continue to pour the solution over the leg. Do not let the cloth dry.
- It is best to fan-dry the leg and foot (especially in patients with mossy foot) after very gently towel-drying.
- Your patient's nails may look brown from using potassium permanganate. This colour disappears when the patient stops using the antiseptic.

2.2. Medicated Creams

If potassium permanganate does not heal entry lesions in deep skin folds, or if the patient has infected wounds, medicated creams will be necessary. Small amounts of medicated cream should be rubbed into the skin at the site of the lesion, until the cream disappears. For severe lesions between the toes or fingers, this process may need to be repeated two times a day.

The availability and cost of antifungal and antibacterial creams vary in different regions, and the medical officer or nurse in charge of the lymphoedema treatment

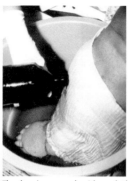

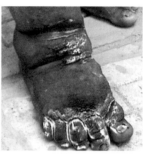

Fig. 4.29 The leg is covered with a cloth soaked in potassium permanganate solution. The health care worker then pours the antiseptic over the leg.

Fig. 4.30 Excessive medicated cream, which is wasteful and ineffective. Teach your patients to use small amounts of medicated cream, and to rub it into the skin until the cream disappears.

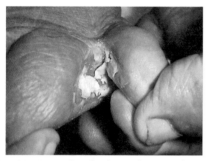

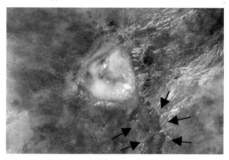

Fig. 4.31 Severe fungal infection between the toes, often found in patients with advanced lymphoedema. The skin is moist and peeling (macerated). Such entry lesions between the toes frequently allow bacteria to enter, resulting in acute attacks.

Fig. 4.32 A skin wound that is infected with bacteria. No pus could be seen at the time this photograph was taken, but the wound is "wet", and excess fluid is draining onto the skin (arrows).

programme will recommend the most suitable ones. Antifungal and antibacterial creams may be purchased separately, or, in some places, combination cream is available. If both types of cream are necessary but combination cream cannot be found, antifungal and antibacterial creams can be mixed and applied together in the same proportion.

2.2.1. Antifungal creams

If fungal infections are found at the site of any entry lesion (and this is very common between the toes), they should be treated with an antifungal cream or solution.

Fungal cream must be rubbed in well (until the cream disappears) at the site of the fungal infection and onto the surrounding skin. Usually, fungal infections between toes must be treated daily for several weeks. Even after apparent cure, daily application of the cream should be continued for at least one week. Teach your patients not to leave excess cream on the skin. Using too much cream is a common mistake; this wastes cream and attracts dirt (Fig. 4.30).

> **Tips for recognizing fungal infections**
> The skin (especially in deep folds and in the spaces between the toes) may:
> - change colour (usually become white or pink) (Figs. 4.24 and 4.25)
> - become broken and cracked
> - become dry and scaly
> - become moist and soft (macerated) (Fig. 4.31)
> - itch or become tender
>
> Some fungal infections are symptomless.

2.2.2. Antibacterial creams

Antibacterial cream is used to treat bacteria-infected entry lesions (Fig. 4.26) in order to prevent acute attacks.

As with fungal cream, antibacterial cream must be rubbed into the affected area well. Cream is usually applied to bacteria-infected entry lesions twice daily until the signs of infection have resolved.

> **Tips for recognizing bacteria-infected wounds**
> - Pus is present (Fig. 4.26).
> - Fever may or may not be present, depending on whether the infection is localized or systemic.
> - Increased wetness. The sudden appearance of significantly increased amounts of exudate (moisture) in a wound (Fig. 4.32) may indicate infection. Some wounds, such as venous ulcers (see chapter 7), tend to be moist, even in the absence of infection. So, infected wounds are usually wet, although not all wet wounds are infected.
> - Increased pain. Usually, increased pain is an indicator that the condition of the wound is worsening. Pain may be a sign that the wound has become infected, although great care should be taken to exclude other causes, especially if the pain is severe and the patient has underlying diseases such diabetes or disease of the arteries or veins. Refer these patients to the clinic for further evaluation.
> - Change in the appearance of the wound. In addition to increased wetness, the infected wound may appear darker in colour and have a tendency to bleed more easily.
> - Odour. The presence of any offensive odour or a change in quality of the odour of a wound may signal infection. Patients with skin lesions caused by certain types of cancer (e.g., malignant fungating lesions) may have a very foul smelling odour. These patients should be referred to a hospital promptly.
> - Abscess. Some infected wounds develop abscesses, localized collections of pus under the skin. If the abscess does not drain on its own, it may be necessary to drain it surgically. These patients should be referred to a clinic or to someone with the proper training to drain the abscess (Fig. 4.33).

Factors related to risk of wound infection

As a health care provider, you should be familiar with factors that increase the risk of bacterial wound infection, such as lack of personal hygiene, shaving, and putting things on the wound that are not clean, such as sand or mud. Certain cultural practices contribute to increased risk of wound infection, and these vary from one place to another. Other risk factors are more universal, but are more difficult to manage: old age, prolonged stay in the hospital, the presence of infection elsewhere in the body, obesity, and underlying diseases, such as diabetes.

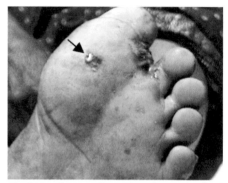

Fig. 4.33 Abscess. The patient has a localized swelling of the sole of the foot, and pus can be seen draining from the abscess onto the skin (arrow).

Growth of bacteria at the site of the wound can be reduced by:

- Good hygiene, not only at the site of the wound, but for the rest of the body as well
- Keeping the wound dry (except while washing)
- Keeping the affected area open to the air

Healing of the wound can be promoted by:

- proper treatment of infection
- controlling bleeding
- avoiding dressings, unless necessary
- not putting ice on an entry lesion
- removing any foreign bodies
- avoiding trauma to the wound
- keeping insects away from the wound

Warning! *Keep all supplies for treating entry lesions out of the reach of children. Potassium permanganate solution has a pleasant purple colour that may attract children, but if swallowed it can be harmful. It must be kept away from children.*

TIPS FOR HYGIENE AND SKIN CARE

- Repeat the washing until the rinse water is clear (Figs. 4.34 and 4.35).
- Usually the first week of hygiene is the most difficult for the patient. After the first week, the time required to wash the legs will decrease, and less water will be required.
- Tell your patients with advanced disease that hygiene gets easier with time.

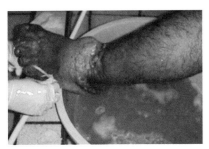

Fig. 4.34 The first wash. Notice the dark colour of the dirty water after the first washing of this patient's leg.

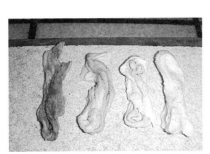

Fig. 4.35 Wash until the rinse water is clear. These pieces of cloth were used in sequence (from left to right) to wash a patient's leg at the time of her first visit to the health worker. Each time the wash basin was emptied and refilled with clean water, a new cloth was used. The patient's leg was washed four times before the health worker declared that the leg was clean.

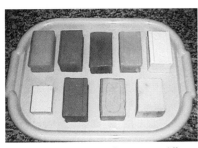

Fig. 4.36 Which soap is best? Many different soaps are available, some better than others. If you do not know which soap to recommend, have your patients use a soap that they are already familiar with. Don't leave the legs unwashed just because you don't know what soap is "best" in your area!

- Remember to wash both legs. It may be easier to remember to wash the normal leg if it is washed first. However, in areas where water supply is limited or if the patient is in a hurry, the diseased leg can be washed first. Regardless of which leg is washed first, advise the patient to look for entry lesions in both the healthy and the affected legs.

- If *both* legs are affected, wash the leg with more advanced lymphoedema first because it will take more time and require more attention.

- If antiseptics or medicated creams are not available, a final light soaping can be left in the deep skin fold or wounds, and the skin dried as described above.

- For patients with early-stage lymphoedema (e.g., stages 1–4) the first treatment for entry lesions, especially fungal infections between the toes, is to wash and dry them well. If no improvement is seen with hygiene in 5 to 7 days, antifungal cream will usually be necessary. There are exceptions to this general rule; for example if your patient has diabetes, antifungal cream should be applied as soon as entry lesions are identified (see chapter 7 for more information). In patients with more advanced lymphoedema (stages 5–7), fungal infections usually require prompt treatment with antifungal creams.

- If fungal entry lesions persist despite hygiene and antifungal treatment, the patient may need to use another kind of cream that contains steroids, which should be used along with the antifungal cream. A medical officer can provide you with more information about steroid creams and when they should be used.

- What kind of soap is best? (Fig. 4.36). There is no specific soap that is best for all filariasis-endemic areas. In general, inexpensive, unscented soap is best. In addition to affordability and other characteristics, a suitable soap will have four qualities: it lasts a long time; it lathers easily; it does not require much water to be rinsed from the skin; and it does not dry the skin. The capacity of soap to produce lather or foam will decrease with the "hardness" of the water, but this should not discourage patients in areas with hard water from practicing hygiene.

• In cases of advanced lymphoedema, adequate hygiene is only possible if the patient has a helper. The helper can wash places that are difficult for the patient to reach. The helper can be a friend or family member.

• Sometimes helpers cannot be found. Together with your patients, you can develop creative ways to improve hygiene. For example, a patient in Recife, Brazil, designed a device to help her wash, dry (Fig. 4.37), and rub cream between her toes.

• Wearing rubber gloves or using a thin plastic bag can help the fingers slide between the deep skin folds. Unless the patient has other diseases that can be spread by touch, gloves are not necessary to prevent infection. Usually, if the patients have not been in the hospital, the bacteria on the skin of the patients are the same as those found on the skin of people without lymphoedema. If you have any doubt about whether gloves are needed, ask the medical officer or a doctor or nurse.

• Advise your patients to avoid keeping their feet wet for long periods of time, for example, when washing clothes (Fig. 4.38). In contrast, wetting the feet and legs for a short time just before the daily hygiene is a good practice.

• Entry lesions may attract flies. Special attention is required for lesions or wounds on the surface of the skin, especially in patients with stage 6 or 7 lymphoedema. Keep these lesions covered with a light cloth or gauze to keep the flies from laying their eggs on the skin (See chapter 8).

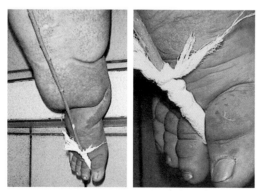

Fig. 4.37 Be creative! Is there no helper available? This patient, who lives alone, found a way to attach small pieces of cloth to a stick to help wash between her toes. With the aid of her health worker, she learned how to use this simple device efficiently without causing harm (for example, scratching the skin). Encourage your patients to work with you to overcome problems creatively.

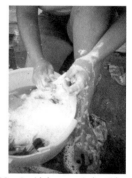

Fig. 4.38 Avoid long periods with wet feet. Wetness promotes the growth of fungi. If your patients' work exposes their feet to water (for example, if they wash lots of clothes), try to find ways to help them protect their feet from being wet for long periods. On the other hand, getting the feet wet just before hygiene can be encouraged—it can make cleaning easier.

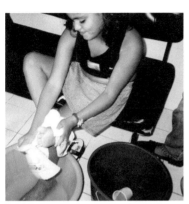

Fig. 4.39 A healthy child practicing hygiene of the leg after learning it from the health worker.

• The best barriers to infection are intact skin and good personal hygiene. In some filariasis-endemic areas, traditional healers will cut the skin of patients with lymphoedema in an attempt to release the excess fluid. This and other practices that break the skin are dangerous for these patients.

• Advising your patient on washing his or her leg is best done after a good assessment of the overall level of hygiene among the patient and his or her family. This assessment is best done through a home visit, where you can examine the living area and inspect the kitchen and bathroom.

• In filariasis-endemic areas, hygiene is important for everyone—even those who do not have lymphoedema. Hygiene is so simple that children can learn and practice it (Fig. 4.39). This will prevent them from having entry lesions.

• If it is culturally acceptable, the affected limbs should not be shaved with a razor. Rather, hair should be cut short with clean scissors.

STEP 3. ELEVATION

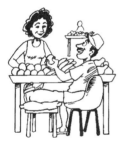

Fig. 4.40 Elevation of the leg while sitting. A pillow supports the leg from the knee to the foot.

Elevation is important for patients with lymphoedema of the leg, particularly when the lymphoedema is complicated by venous insufficiency (see chapter 7). Elevation helps to prevent fluid from accumulating in the leg, which can lead to worsening of the lymphoedema. For patients to receive the full benefit when they elevate their legs, the correct position is very important (Fig. 4.40), especially for large, heavy legs.

Sitting

1. Raise both legs, if possible, always in a comfortable position. Ideally, raise the feet to almost as high as the hips. If this is not comfortable (it may not be for patients with advanced lymphoedema), raise the feet as high as is comfortable.

2. Always bend the knee slightly; a thin pillow should be placed under the knee for support.

3. The lower leg should be well supported on a stool or chair.

4. Avoid any pressure on the ankle. If the pillow creates pressure on the ankle, extend the ankle beyond the pillow.

5. If any pain or discomfort develops, change position.

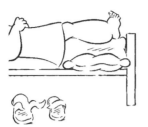

Fig. 4.41 The correct way to elevate the leg while sleeping. The pillow (or other object) used to elevate the foot of the bed is placed under the mattress, not on top.

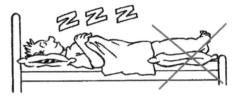

Fig. 4.42 If the pillow is placed on top of the mattress, the leg may fall off while the patient is sleeping. If this happens, the patient does not benefit from elevation of the leg.

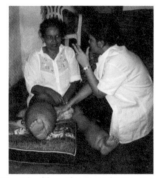

Fig. 4.43 A health worker is explaining to a patient the right way to exercise while sitting on the ground. For comfort and support, place a thin pillow under the leg, including the knee. It is best to rest the back against a wall.

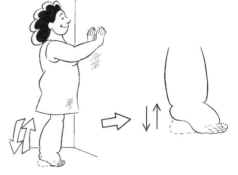

Fig. 4.44 "Up on the toes" exercise, with the hands against the wall for support.

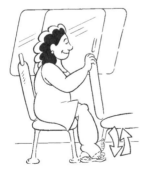

Fig. 4.45 This patient practices her "toe point exercise" while on the bus.

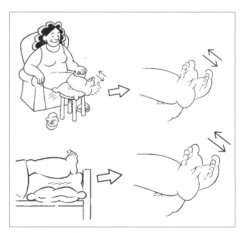

Fig. 4.46 The "toe point exercise" while sitting or lying down.

> **Warning!**
> - Do not use supports with sharp edges that put pressure on, or dig into, the elevated leg.
> - Avoid sitting with the legs crossed at the knees.

Lying down

1. Elevate the foot of the bed
2. Place a support (bricks, pillows, etc.) under the mattress to raise the foot of the bed evenly.
3. The heel of the patient's foot should be a little higher than the level of the heart (Fig. 4.41).
4. Place a pillow under the knees to bend the knees slightly.
5. Raise the entire leg, not just the foot. For example, placing a pillow directly under the foot is incorrect (Fig. 4.42). The foot can fall off the pillow during the night, and the benefit of elevation will not occur.

> **Warning!** *Patients with heart problems and shortness of breath should not elevate their legs, unless advised by a doctor.*

STEP 4. EXERCISE

Exercise is useful for patients with lymphoedema. In general, the more patients exercise, the more they benefit. They can exercise anywhere and at any time. However, patients should never exercise during an acute attack (see chapter 5).

Besides walking short distances for exercise, patients can do specific exercises explained below. There are four positions for doing leg exercises: sitting on the ground (Fig. 4.43), sitting on a chair, standing, or lying down.

"Up on the toes" exercise (this is also called the "ballerina exercise" in Brazil.)
- Stand on both feet with feet slightly apart, holding on to a person or other type of support (Fig. 4.44).
- Rise up on to the toes of both feet at the same time, and then sink back down onto flat feet.
- Repeat 5–15 times, or as many times as comfortable.
- If the patient is unable to rise up on both feet at the same time, this exercise can be done one foot at a time.

"Toe point" exercise
- While sitting or lying down, point toes towards the floor (Figs. 4.45 and 4.46).
- Then point the toes (flex the ankle) upwards.

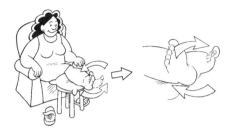

Fig. 4.47 Practicing the "circle exercise" while sitting, rotating both to the right and the left.

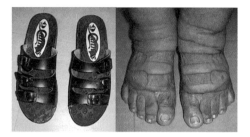

Fig. 4.48 Tight shoes. An example of shoes that are unsuitable for this patient. Such tight shoes can easily produce entry lesions.

a   b   c   d   e

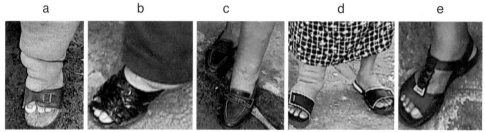

Fig. 4.49 Patients with various stages of lymphoedema, with inappropriate (a and b) and appropriate shoes (c, d, and e).

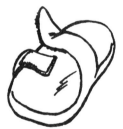

Fig. 4.50 An example of a shoe suitable for patients with lymphoedema. Other styles can also be developed according to the stage and severity of lymphoedema.

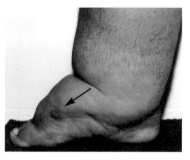

Fig. 4.51 A blister (arrow) that developed when this patient wore uncomfortable tennis shoes.

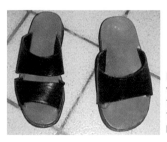

Fig. 4.52 Be creative! You and your patients can work with a local shoemaker to develop shoes that both protect the feet of your patients and are stylish and attractive. These sandals are the result of one such partnership.

- Repeat 5–15 times, or as many times as comfortable.
- Repeat with the other leg.
- This exercise can also be done while standing if the patient does not have advanced disease.

"Circle" exercise
- While sitting or laying down, point the big toe and move the foot in a circular motion, both to the right (clockwise) and to the left (counter clockwise) (Fig. 4.47).
- Repeat with the other leg.
- If sitting on the floor, protect the heel with a flat pillow.
- This exercise can also be done while standing if the patient does not have advanced disease.

STEP 5. WEARING SHOES

Shoes protect feet from injury. Protecting the bottom of the feet is very important. For some patients, protecting the sides and top of the feet is also important. Patients should avoid shoes that make their feet hot and sweaty, or that are too tight (Fig. 4.48).

What kind of shoes? (Fig. 4.49)

Shoes should
- protect the feet from injury
- protect the feet from dirt on the ground
- be comfortable (not too tight)
- allow air around the feet
- have low heels, if any.

Canvas or cloth shoes allow more air to circulate around the feet than plastic or leather shoes.

Sandals are better than closed shoes for most patients (Fig. 4.50). Patients with early-stage lymphoedema may be able to wear closed shoes.

Do not wear shoes that cause blisters (Fig. 4.51) or sore places on the feet. These blisters may cause entry lesions, which can lead to acute attacks. If blisters do occur, hygiene is especially important. Do not pop the blisters.

Avoid shoes that make the feet hot and sweaty or that do not fit correctly (Fig. 4.48).

You and your patients may need to be creative to find the right shoes or to modify shoes, with the help of a cobbler (shoe-maker), to fit properly (Fig. 4.52).

STEP 6. ADJUNCT MEASURES

6.1. Emollients (moisturising agents)

As a general rule, humidity tends to be high in tropical areas where lymphatic filariasis occurs, and dry skin is not a common problem. However, skin that is too dry can increase the risk of entry lesions. Dry skin can be treated and prevented with emollients, which are moisturizing agents that are applied to the skin. Several types of emollient are available, including bath oils, soap substitutes, lotions, creams, and ointments.

We do not advise the routine use of emollients for lymphoedema treatment and prevention in filariasis-endemic area, although they may be recommended for individual patients. Emollients should be avoided on wet lesions. They should not be used on mossy lesions, in deep skin folds, or between the toes. Lanolin is a good emollient, but it can be contaminated with substances that cause allergic reactions when applied to the skin. Therefore, patients in filariasis-endemic areas should generally avoid products that contain lanolin.

6.2. Compressive measures—bandaging

Bandaging, when indicated and used correctly by individual patients, can provide good short-term results. With bandaging, the legs may become smaller more quickly, but there are several disadvantages to bandaging:

- Proper bandages are very expensive and hard to keep clean.
- Bandages can be hot or uncomfortable, and can cause itching.
- Bandages can keep patients from exercising.
- It may take many clinic visits for patients to learn how put on the bandages correctly. Some patients will always need help from a skilled person to put on the bandages properly.
- Applying bandages properly can take a lot of time.

If bandages are not put on correctly:
- Uneven or excessive pressure can damage the lymphatic vessels, which can worsen, rather than improve, the condition of the leg.
- If bandages are placed over an entry lesion, they can cause pain and keep it from healing.
- Using bandages too soon after an acute attack, while there is still some inflammation, may damage the lymphatics and the skin.
- If use of the bandages is stopped, swelling of the leg may return rapidly, even in the absence of an acute attack. This can be discouraging for patients.

For these reasons, bandaging is not recommended as a public health measure for patients with lymphoedema. For certain individual patients, if resources are available, bandages may be used, but they should be used with care. If bandages are used:

- Cotton or other soft material should be placed in the folds, especially in the deep folds, to avoid uneven compression and damage to the lymphatics.
- Bandages should be put on first thing in the morning and taken off at night.
- Bandages should be kept clean.
- Old bandages should be replaced with new ones at regular intervals, as needed.

Warning! Bandages should never be used during an acute attack.

6.3. Other compressive measures

In addition to bandaging, other compressive garments, such as stockings, are available.

Compared to bandages, stockings have certain advantages:

- They make it easier for the patient to exercise
- They may be easier and take less time to put on and take off
- They are thinner and more comfortable
- Special training is not necessary to use compressive garments. The patient just has to learn how to put them on and take them off.

However, they:

- are expensive and need to be replaced often
- often must be specially fitted to the patient's leg
- can be hard to keep clean

Notice: Compressive measures can be very important for patients with venous insufficiency (see Chapter 7).

6.4. Other physical measures for lymphoedema management

In developed countries with considerable resources, some patients with lymphoedema benefit from breathing exercises and gentle massage. Breathing exercises can be done at home by the patient and are therefore inexpensive. In contrast, proper lymphoedema massage requires special techniques and training, and may therefore be more costly, as well as time-consuming. In this book, neither of these two measures is recommended for lymphoedema management in the context of public health programs in filariasis-endemic areas. However, both measures may be helpful for individual patients. They can be used if resources and health workers with the appropriate training and expertise are available.

6.5. Prophylactic antibiotics

The use of hygiene, antiseptics, and medicated creams will decrease the frequency of acute attacks in all patients. In patients with early stage lymphoedema, these measures will prevent acute attacks. Patients with more advanced lymphoedema and

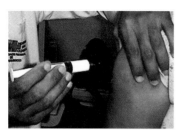

Fig. 4.53 A patient receiving an antibiotic injection in the clinic.

many entry lesions, however, may continue to have some acute attacks. If acute attacks continue, it may be necessary for the patient to take antibiotics prophylactically (as a preventive measure), to help prevent bacterial infections. Antibiotics can be given by mouth or by injection, the latter usually every three weeks (Fig. 4.53). Thus, patients who continue to have repeated acute attacks, in spite of hygiene and skin care, should be referred to a doctor, who can evaluate the patient and prescribe the right antibiotics.

Important: If a patient has stage 6 or 7 lymphoedema and very severe entry lesions, prophylactic antibiotics may be advised before washing the leg for the first time and for the following 5 days. For such patients, consult a physician to determine whether prophylactic antibiotics are needed. If so, they should be started at least 24 hours before the first washing.

6.6. Cosmetic surgery

Your patients may ask you about surgery as an option for treatment. Surgery to remove the swelling of the leg is not appropriate as a public health measure: it is expensive, difficult, and often the results are not satisfactory. However, cosmetic surgery, to remove knobs, help improve the appearance of the skin, or decrease the possibility of trauma and potential entry lesions, may be recommended for the individual patient (Fig. 4.54). This surgery is usually done in an outpatient clinic. Before surgery can be considered, however, the patient should be under treatment, and should not have had acute attacks for several months. If you think your patients may benefit from cosmetic surgery, you can refer them to a hospital or clinic for consultation.

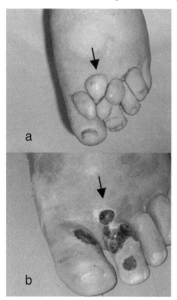

Fig. 4.54 Cosmetic surgery. Surgery to remove knobs (arrows) can benefit some patients, as shown for this patient before (upper) and after (lower) surgery. The removal of the knobs reduces the risk of trauma, and makes it easier to find a suitable, comfortable shoe.

For a few patients, lymphoedema may improve so much that they develop redundant or loose skin, sometimes called "bag leg". These patients can eventually benefit from cosmetic surgery, in which the surgeon removes the excess skin. However, to avoid acute attacks, it is important that the patient be well adapted and motivated to continue with good lymphoedema management. If acute attacks occur after such cosmetic surgery, the consequences may be very serious for the patient.

DEVELOPING A PATIENT MANAGEMENT PLAN

The basic principles of lymphoedema management are the same for all patients, but the degree and intensity with which they must practice each of them depends largely on the stage of lymphoedema. The following table outlines the recommended management for each stage of lymphoedema.

LYMPHOEDEMA MANAGEMENT, BY STAGE — A GENERAL GUIDE

Treatment Component	Stage 1	Stage 2	Stage 3	Stage 4	Stage 5	Stage 6	Stage 7
Hygiene (washing and drying)	Yes (ideally at night)	Yes (ideally at night)	Yes (ideally at night)	Yes (ideally at night)	Yes (twice a day if possible)	Yes (twice a day if possible)	Yes (twice a day if possible)
Care of entry lesions	If present	If present	If present	If present	If present	If present	If present
Exercise	Yes	Yes	Yes	Yes	If possible	If possible	If possible
Elevation	Usually not necessary	At night	Day and night	Day and night	Day and night	Day and night if possible	Day and night if possible
Prophylactic creams	No	No	Usually not necessary	Usually not necessary	Usually necessary	Necessary	Necessary
Prophylatic systemic antibiotics (send to doctor)	No	No	No	Usually not necessary	Usually necessary (if acute attacks persist)	Necessary	Necessary
Cosmetic surgery	Not applicable	Not applicable	Not applicable	If medically indicated	If medically indicated	If medically indicated	If medically indicated

Recommended Reading

Addiss DG, Dreyer G. Treatment of Lymphatic Filariasis. In: *Lymphatic Filariasis*, Nutman TB (ed). London: Imperial College Press. 2000; 151–199.

Campisi C. A rational approach to the management of lymphedema. *Lymphology* 1991; 24:48–53, 1991.

Dreyer G, Medeiros Z, Netto MJ, Leal NC, DeCastro LG, Piessens WF. Acute attacks in the extremities of persons living in an area endemic for bancroftian filariasis: differentiation of two syndromes. *Trans Roy Soc Trop Med Hyg* 1999; 93:413–417.

Dreyer G, Piessens W. Worms and microorganisms can cause lymphatic disease in residents of filariasis-endemic areas. In: *Lymphatic Filariasis*, Nutman TB (ed). London: Imperial College Press. 2000; 245–264.

Morison M, Moffatt C, Bridel-Nixon J, Bale S. *Nursing Management of Chronic Wounds* 1997; Mosby, London.

Shenoy RK, Sandhya K, Suma TK, Kumaraswami V. A preliminary study of filariasis related to acute lymphangitis with special reference to precipitating factors and treatment modalities. *Southeast Asian J Trop Med Pub Health* 1995; 26:301–305.

Shenoy RK, Suma TK, Rajan K, Kumaraswami V. Prevention of acute lymphangitis in brugian filariasis: comparison of the efficacy of ivermectin and diethylcarbamazine, each combined with local treatment of the affected limb. *Ann Trop Med Parasitol* 1998; 92:587–594.

Recommended Viewing

Lymphatic Filariasis: Hope for a better life. (Training video). Program for patients, 21 minutes. Program for health care workers, 58 minutes.

For further information on the scientific publications please contact a university or medical school library, or write to Centers for Disease Control and Prevention (contact information on page 111).

Copies of the video may be purchased through the Public Health Foundation in the United States (contact information on page 111).

CHAPTER FIVE
Assessment and Management of Acute Attacks

Patients with damaged lymphatic vessels and lymphoedema usually have small cuts, breaks, or scratches in the skin and between the toes, called "entry lesions". Lesions between the toes present the greatest risk of acute attacks. Lesions in deep folds and small lesions on the skin surface are considered moderate risk, while cracks in the sole of the foot and uncomplicated onychomycosis are associated with a low risk. Entry lesions allow bacteria to enter the skin, and they multiply quickly. Large numbers of bacteria cause the inflammation that is characteristic of an acute attack (Figs. 5.01). The skin becomes painful, warm, swollen, and red, and the patient develops a fever, headache, chills and sometimes nausea and vomiting. Some patients will develop blisters (Fig. 5.02). Occasionally, bacteria get into the blood and may cause a life-threatening illness. This can be a problem in elderly people, who can be very sick but may not have obvious signs of severe illness, such as high fever.

Acute Attack Assessment

In many patients, the first sign of an acute attack in the leg is an enlarged, tender, and painful lymph node in the inguinal area. Afterwards, inflammation appears in the leg with or without anterograde lymphangitis, that is, inflammation of the lymphatic vessel that begins in the limbs and progresses towards the trunk or centre of the body. Most patients will have three to five days of redness, severe pain, and swelling. Your patients may tell you that they could not walk or get out of bed. Sometimes the skin is so tender that it will hurt even when a breeze blows across the leg.

Even if you do not see the patient during an acute attack, in addition to the description of his or her symptoms, certain physical signs will tell you that the patient

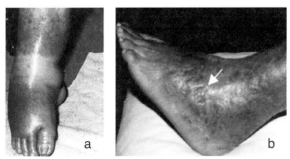

Fig. 5.01 Two examples of an acute attack. The patient on the left has entry lesions between the toes (not shown). The patient on the right has an entry lesion on the foot (arrow).

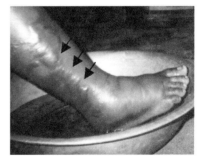

Fig. 5.02 Blisters. Some patients develop blisters during an acute attack. The blisters are very painful and can worsen the course of an acute attack (for example, they can become infected). Note how shiny the skin is.

recently had an acute attack. For example, after an acute attack, dry, peeling skin is commonly seen (Fig. 5.03). After the acute attack subsides, the patient may develop darkening of the skin in the area where the attack occurred (Fig. 5.04). It may take a long time for the skin to return to its original colour.

Acute attacks always make lymphoedema worse. If your patients can prevent acute attacks, they can prevent elephantiasis and keep their disease from getting worse.

Acute Attack Management

The first step in managing an acute attack is to relieve pain.

Relieve pain – Cool the leg

- Apply a clean cloth compress soaked with water at room temperature or slightly cooler. The compress should go all away around the leg (Fig. 5.05). Put plastic under the leg to keep the bed or chair dry.

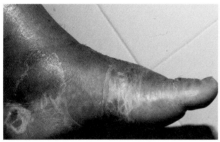

Fig. 5.03 Peeling skin—a sign of a recent acute attack.

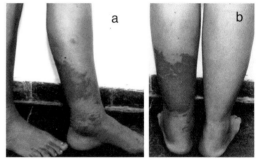

Fig. 5.04 a, b Hyperpigmentation, or darkening of the skin. Hyperpigmentation occurs after an acute attack, even when there are no blisters. A view from the side (a), and from the back (b). In this patient, lymphoedema persisted after the acute attack, and became chronic.

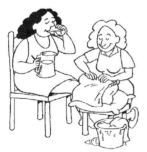

Fig. 5.05 Apply a cool compress to relieve pain during an acute attack. Use water at room temperature or a little bit cooler. Change the compress when it gets warm.

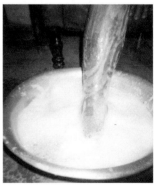

Fig. 5.06 Washing during an acute attack. The patient should begin to wash the leg again as soon as she or he begins to feel better. The patient should look for the entry lesions and be sure to wash them well.

- Change the compress when it becomes warm. A fan placed near the compress will help keep it cooler. The compress should not get dry.
- The patient can also soak the leg in a tub or bucket filled with cool water if she or he has nobody to help change the compress.
- Cool the leg until the pain goes away. If "hot and cold" theories of disease are part of your culture, then be sure you address this issue with the patient and stress that water at room temperature or cooler is needed for the "hot" leg or affected area.

Alert: If you use cold water, it should be only a little cooler than room temperature. Iced water can damage the skin.

Rest and elevation
- Rest and elevate the leg comfortably as much as possible.
- Exercise is painful. Do not exercise during an acute attack.

Other measures for managing acute attacks
Medicine for fever. Give the patient medicine for fever as necessary (e.g., paracetomol). Aspirin should not be given in areas where dengue is common, unless prescribed by a doctor. It is recommended that medication be taken every 6 hours until the fever lessens.

Drink lots of water or fruit juices.

Systemic antibiotics (oral or injectable). Antibiotics can shorten the attack and help prevent further skin damage. Antibiotics are recommended if a doctor or nurse can see the patient, the antibiotics are available, and the patient can afford them.

Notice: During the first 24 hours the pain may be very severe. Do not try to look for entry lesions between the toes if the acute attack involves the foot or toes.

Notice: Most patients can easily care for their acute attacks at home. The patient should cool the leg as soon as an acute attack starts. This helps to prevent further skin damage.

Hygiene and treatment of entry lesions
Hygiene is very important. Patients should follow these steps during an acute attack as soon as the pain lessens.

- After washing the hands well (both the patient and any helpers), wash the leg with soap and clean water, but much more gently and more carefully than ususal (Fig. 5.06)
- Dry the leg, much more gently and carefully than usual.
- Identify and care for any entry lesions.
  - Apply an antiseptic to the skin.
  - Apply medicated cream to any entry lesions.

Danger signs

If your patients have any of the problems listed below during acute attack, a doctor or nurse should see them.

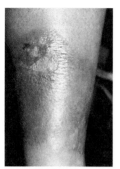

- Very high fever, confusion, headache, drowsiness, or vomiting
- Fever, shaking, chills, or pain in the leg that do not respond to treatment within 24 hours
- Splitting of the skin because of a rapid increase in the size of the leg
- Pus in the affected area (Fig. 5.07)
- Progression of the redness, pain, and swelling in the leg despite appropriate treatment
- Other signs or symptoms that you are not familiar with and that you think may need special attention

Fig. 5.07 Appearance of pus during an acute attack. If the skin cracks during an acute attack and pus is visible, you should refer the patient to a doctor or nurse. She or he may need medical care.

Systemic antibiotics and other measures, including staying in the hospital overnight, may be necessary for these patients. Although rare, patients have died from acute attacks.

People who require special attention

The following groups of people should see a doctor or nurse when they have an acute attack, even if they do not have the problems listed above.

- The elderly, especially if they do not have a high fever during the acute attack, seem to have no energy, and don't care for food or drink
- Alcoholics
- Pregnant women and children who do not improve within 24 hours
- Malnourished patients
- People with other chronic diseases, such as heart and lung problems, high blood pressure, or diabetes (see chapter 7)

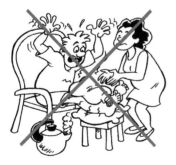

Fig. 5.08 Do not apply anything warm or hot to the leg during an acute attack.

Harmful practices

In every country with filariasis, people have ways to deal with acute attacks. Some of these treatments may help, others make no difference, and others are harmful. Examples of practices that should be discouraged because they are harmful include:

- Putting anything that is warm or hot on the skin (Fig. 5.08)
- Cutting the skin to remove excess fluid or blood

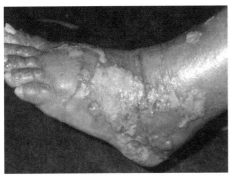

Fig. 5.09 Infected blisters, with pus. Blisters frequently become infected when they rupture or are popped. They are extremely painful. The patient may need to be referred to a doctor or nurse in order to manage the pain and the infection.

- Bandaging the leg
- Rubbing herbs, ashes, or anything unclean onto the skin
- Popping, opening, or cutting blisters (Fig. 5.09)
- Burying the leg in the ground
- Actively peeling off the skin that begins to peel on its own after the acute attack.

Do not peel off the skin; rather, let it come off on its own. To reduce the possibility of trauma and further damage, however, the health worker can carefully remove excess peeled skin with clean scissors. Patients may be able to do this as well, if they are properly instructed and trained by the health worker.

Tips for acute attack management

- If the mother feels that she is able, it is OK for her to breastfeed during an acute attack—this will not hurt the baby or the mother (Fig. 5.10).
- The acute attack is not contagious. Do not be afraid to touch the patient. It is good practice to wash your hands afterwards.
- Once the acute attack subsides, you should talk with your patient about what factors may have led to the acute attack and help your patient to overcome them. We highlight the following such factors:
  - Finding clean water may be difficult.
  - Lack of time for washing every day.
  - Patients may feel that hygiene is too simple a solution, and some may want more dramatic or more rapid medical treatment.
  - Recognizing hidden or small entry lesions can be difficult.
  - Some patients may not be able to afford some or all of the supplies needed to treat entry lesions.
  - Lack of knowledge regarding hygiene and skin care.
  - Some patients cannot afford specially fitted shoes.
  - Lack of a skilled shoemaker who can make simple, protective shoes to fit large feet.
  - Some patients may need help and do not have someone to wash their leg.
  - Lack of motivation for hygiene because of other urgent and personal problems (e.g., death or illness in the family).
  - Poor personal hygiene (e.g., dirty clothes, hands).

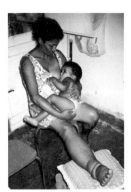

Fig. 5.10 May I feed my baby during an acute attack? Yes—it is OK for your patient to breastfeed during an acute attack, if she feels well enough. Remind her to sit comfortably, with the leg elevated, or to lie in bed.

Acute attacks and success of lymphoedema management

The frequency of acute attacks is one of the most important indicators of success or failure of your program. Frequency of acute attacks can therefore be used as a powerful monitoring tool.

An additional indicator of program success is the decreasing frequency of entry lesions in your patients, especially entry lesions between the toes, since the presence of entry lesions is a risk factor for acute attacks.

An example of a form that can be used to monitor progress in your patients is shown in the Appendix, page 89. This form can be modified to meet the needs of health workers in different filariasis-endemic areas.

Recommended Reading

Addiss DG, Dreyer G. Treatment of Lymphatic Filariasis. In: *Lymphatic Filariasis,* Nutman TB (ed). London: Imperial College Press. 2000; 151–199.

Dreyer G, Medeiros Z, Netto MJ, Leal NC, DeCastro LG, Piessens WF. Acute attacks in the extremities of persons living in an area endemic for bancroftian filariasis: differentiation of two syndromes. *Trans Roy Soc Trop Med Hyg* 1999; 93:413–417.

Dreyer G, Piessens W. Worms and microorganisms can cause lymphatic disease in residents of filariasis-endemic areas. In: *Lymphatic Filariasis,* Nutman TB (ed). London: Imperial College Press. 2000; 245-264.

Shenoy RK, Sandhya K, Suma TK, Kumaraswami V. A preliminary study of filariasis related to acute lymphangitis with special reference to precipitating factors and treatment modalities. *Southeast Asian J Trop Med Pub Health* 1995; 26:301–305.

Recommended Viewing

Lymphatic Filariasis: Hope for a better life. (Training video). Program for patients, 21 minutes. Program for health care workers, 58 minutes.

For further information on the scientific publications please contact a university or medical school library, or write to Centers for Disease Control and Prevention (contact information on page 111).

Copies of the video may be purchased through the Public Health Foundation in the United States (contact information on page 111).

CHAPTER SIX
Urogenital Problems in Filariasis

As you have learned, filariasis causes problems in the legs, arms, and breasts. Filariasis also causes chronic genital problems (in the penis, scrotum, and tissues inside the scrotum), and chronic urinary tract problems. Men with filariasis most often develop genital problems, while urinary tract problems affect both men and women. These problems have a huge emotional and social impact. Treatment varies depending on the type of genital or urinary tract problem. Therefore, correct diagnosis is important.

Genital Problems

In men, lymphatic filariasis can cause the genitals to become enlarged and deformed. Even when men suffer from these problems, they will hide them and you may not be aware of their suffering. They may not mention their problems, but their lives are deeply affected. These men feel ashamed and embarrassed, and they become socially isolated.

This section of the book addresses the different types of genital disease in males and the types of treatment that are available.

The normal appearance of the genitals in adult men is shown in Fig. 6.01. The scrotal sac, a thin sac made of skin and other layers of tissue, covers the testes. The normal size of the scrotum and its contents varies from man to man. The skin of scrotum and penis is normally thin and soft.

In men with lymphatic filariasis, there are two main ways in which the scrotum and its contents become enlarged. First, fluid can collect inside the scrotal sac (Fig. 6.02); and second, the skin can be affected (Fig. 6.03). You need to be able to tell these two conditions apart, because the treatment is different.

Hydrocoele

Collection of fluid inside the scrotal sac is the most common genital problem caused by filariasis. The scrotum becomes enlarged because there is excess liquid inside the scrotal sac, around the testicles. This is known as a hydrocoele. The fluid can collect on only one side (Fig. 6.04) or on both sides (Fig. 6.05).

Hydrocoeles can be small and may hardly be noticed by the patient (Fig. 6.06), or very large, causing a great deal of disability (Fig. 6.07). Hydrocoeles can become so large that the penis becomes hidden (Fig. 6.07 and 6.08).

If a patient has only hydrocoele, the skin of the scrotum and penis is normal—thin and soft (Fig. 6.09).

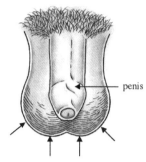

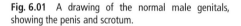

sac of scrotal skin covering the two testes

Fig. 6.01 A drawing of the normal male genitals, showing the penis and scrotum.

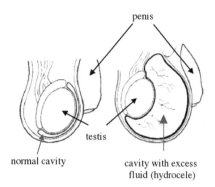

Fig. 6.02 A cross-sectional ("cut-away") view, from the side, of a normal scrotal sac (on the left) and a scrotal sac in which there is excess fluid, or hydrocoele (on the right). The blue arrows indicate the site at which fluid can accumulate inside the scrotal sac, causing hydrocoele.

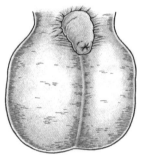

Fig. 6.03 The skin of the penis and scrotum in this patient is thick; he has lymphoedema of the skin of the scrotal sac and penis.

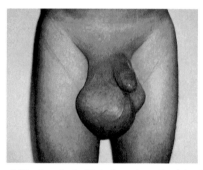

Fig. 6.04 A patient with hydrocoele on the right side. There is no increase in volume on the left side. The skin of the scrotal sac and the penis is normal.

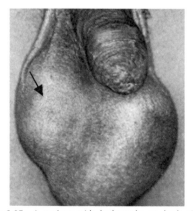

Fig. 6.05 A patient with hydrocoele on both sides (bilateral hydrocoele). The hydrocoele on the right side (arrow) is smaller than the one on the left.

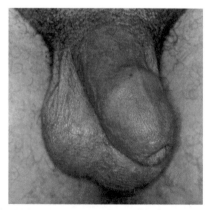

Fig. 6.06 A young man with a small hydrocoele on the left side. The hydrocoele was so small that the patient was not aware that he had it.

Management of Hydrocoele

The good news about hydrocoele is that it can be treated with surgery. This surgery is available in many parts of the world (Fig. 6.10). If your patient seems to have increased volume inside his scrotal sac, you should advise him to see a doctor for two reasons: 1) to discuss the possibility of surgery, and 2) to make sure he does not have other diseases that may be causing increased volume inside the scrotal sac (see chapter 8).

In filariasis-endemic areas, men with hydrocoele frequently have adult filarial worms in their lymphatic vessels. These men should be treated with antifilarial drugs. If your patients with hydrocoele live in a community where there is no program of mass treatment (in which all community members are treated with antifilarial drugs at least once a year), refer them to a doctor, hospital, or clinic where they can be treated with drugs to kill the filarial worms.

Patients with large hydrocoeles may be prone to fungal infections in the contact area between the leg and the scrotum because of moisture. Advise these patients to wash, dry well, and in some cases, use antifungal cream.

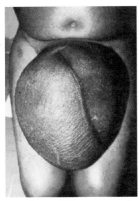

Fig. 6.07 A very large bilateral hydrocoele. The penis is completely hidden. Sexual intercourse and hygiene of the penis are not possible for this patient. He also may have problems urinating.

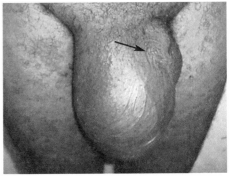

Fig. 6.08 A patient with a moderate unilateral hydrocele and hidden penis (arrow.)

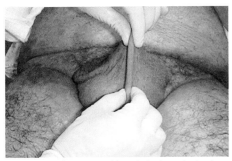

Fig. 6.09 When men with only hydrocoele (and no lymphoedema of the scrotal sac) are examined, the skin feels normal (soft and thin).

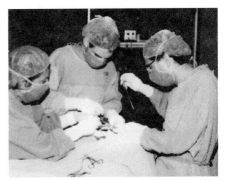

Fig. 6.10 Hydrocoele is a condition that is curable with surgery.

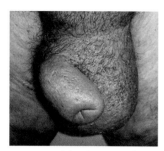

Fig. 6.11 A man with lymphoedema of both the penis and the scrotum.

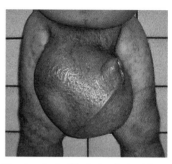

Fig. 6.12 A patient with elephantiasis of the scrotum. Note the deformed shape of the scrotum, which reaches to the man's knees. The penis and midline of the scrotum are displaced to the left. Sexual intercourse is not possible for this man.

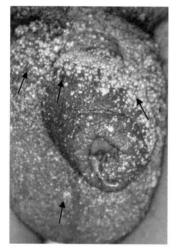

Fig. 6.13 A patient with lymph scrotum. Note the many vesicles on the surface of the skin of the penis and scrotal sac, which are filled with milky white lymph fluid (arrows).

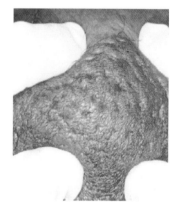

Fig. 6.14 Lymphoedema of the scrotum. On physical examination, the skin is hard and thick.

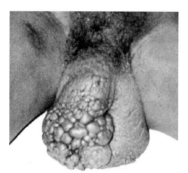

Fig. 6.15 Elephantiasis of the penis, with many knobs. This patient also has lymphoedema of the scrotal sac.

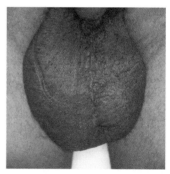

Fig. 6.16 A patient with early lymphoedema of the scrotal sac, photo taken in 1995. The same patient is shown again in Figure 6.17.

Problems Affecting the Skin of the Scrotum and Penis

The skin of the scrotum and penis can be affected by:

- Lymphoedema (fluid inside the skin) (Fig. 6.11)
- Elephantiasis (advanced lymphoedema) (Fig. 6.12)
- Lymph scrotum (vesicles on the skin) (Fig. 6.13)

Lymphoedema and elephantiasis

When the skin of the scrotum is affected by lymphoedema, it becomes thicker and harder than normal and loses its normal texture (Fig. 6.14). Lymphoedema always affects both sides of the scrotum.

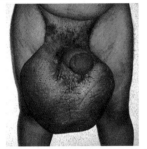

Fig. 6.17 The same patient shown in Figure 6.16. This photo was taken in 1999, after 4 years of repeated bacterial acute attacks. This man now has elephantiasis. This condition could have been prevented if he had avoided the acute attacks through hygiene and skin care.

Lymphoedema of the genitals is not staged like lymphoedema in the leg. However, if the genitals are deformed or very enlarged, and the skin is hard, thick, or has knobs or bumps on the skin, the patient has elephantiasis (Fig. 6.15).

Most commonly, lymphoedema affects the scrotal sac, but the penis may be affected as well. However, lymphoedema only rarely affects just the skin of the penis.

Just as acute attacks cause lymphoedema of the leg to progress to elephantiasis, so do acute attacks in the scrotum or penis (Fig. 6.16 and 6.17).

> *Notice:* As with the limbs or breast, patients who have lymphoedema of the skin of the scrotum or penis, but who have never had an acute attack in this area (so-called "cold lymphoedema") are unlikely to have filarial disease. These patients should be referred to the clinic for further evaluation. These patients will benefit from the hygiene recommended in this book, even though the cause of their lymphoedema is not related to lymphatic filariasis.

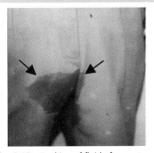

Fig. 6.18 Leaking of fluid after rupture of vesicles in a man with lymph scrotum. Leaking of fluid is unpredictable, and causes the clothes to get wet, leading to embarrassment and shame.

Lymph scrotum

The third skin problem caused by lymphatic filariasis is lymph scrotum (Fig. 6.13). Although the skin changes of lymph scrotum are more common in the scrotal sac, they can also affect the penis. Men with lymph scrotum have vesicles, or small blisters, on the skin of the scrotum or penis. The vesicles are very delicate, and they contain fluid, which may be milky white, straw-coloured, or even pink if blood is present. When they break open, the fluid leaks onto the skin, and the patient's clothes get wet (Fig. 6.18).

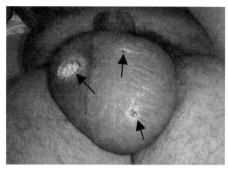

Fig. 6.19 Entry lesions (arrows), in various stages of healing. This patient is recovering from an acute attack. The scrotal sac is still swollen and red.

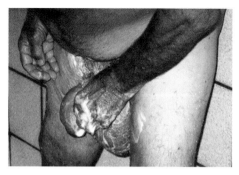

Fig. 6.20 Hygiene. A patient with lymphoedema washing his genital area with soap and water.

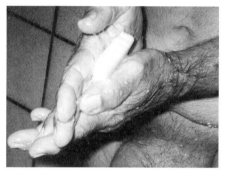

Fig. 6.21 Preparing for hygiene. Before hygiene, the hands should be washed well.

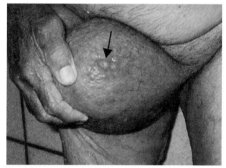

Fig. 6.22 Looking for entry lesions. The patient is instructed how to look for entry lesions (arrow). It may be difficult for men with large-volume lymphoedema to see some entry lesions; they should be taught how to recognize entry lesions by touch in areas that are difficult to see.

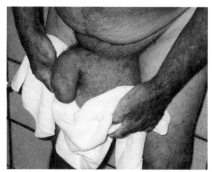

Fig. 6.23 Drying the penis and scrotal sac after washing. This should be done carefully and gently.

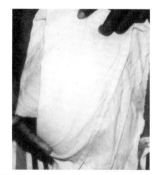

Fig. 6.24 A patient demonstrating the correct way to use a dressing (the white cloth) for his lymph scrotum. After covering the affected area with the dressing, the underwear (with red, white, and blue stripes) is pulled up around the dressing.

For some men with lymph scrotum, the size of the scrotum may be almost normal, but for others, the scrotum becomes very large. Men with lymph scrotum often have frequent acute attacks. These men also develop lymphoedema of the scrotum and penis.

Management of lymphoedema, elephantiasis, and lymph scrotum

You already know that good hygiene helps prevent acute attacks in people with lymphoedema of the legs. Good hygiene is even more important for men with lymphoedema of the scrotum or penis (Fig. 6.19). Encourage these patients to carefully wash their penis, scrotum, and the areas around the scrotum with soap and clean water every day (Fig. 6.20). The water should be at room temperature.

Before washing the genital area, your patients should first wash their hands (Fig 6.21) and then look for entry lesions (Fig. 6.22). Then they should wash the scrotum and penis with soap and water (Fig. 6.20), and dry the area well afterwards (Fig. 6.23).

If they find entry lesions, your patients should use an antibacterial cream after washing and drying. They should rub a small amount of cream into any area with an entry lesion. To avoid breaking the vesicles, men with lymph scrotum should wash and dry very carefully. Even if the vesicles are leaking, the patient should apply cream, gently and carefully.

Men with lymph scrotum often use a dressing or other material, such as a plastic bag, to absorb or collect the fluid. Tell these patients to use a clean dressing made of cloth. The dressing must be changed often and washed well. After washing, it should be dried in the sun, ironed, and stored in a clean place. Tell your patients to cover only the affected area with the dressing (Fig. 6.24), which is placed underneath or inside the underwear. Tight dressings and plastic bags (Fig. 6.25 and 6.26) should be avoided.

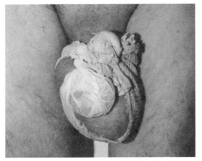

Fig. 6.25 To absorb and collect leaking fluid, this man with lymph scrotum uses a cloth wrapped around the scrotal sac and a plastic bag around the penis.

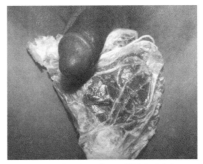

Fig. 6.26 Use of a plastic bag, which is tightly attached to the base of the scrotal sac, to collect milky fluid in a man with lymph scrotum. Tight dressings and plastic bags should be avoided, but if the patient needs to use plastic to collect the fluid, it must be changed as frequently as possible, and should not be applied tightly.

We do not routinely use antiseptic on the skin of the scrotum and penis. This is because the skin in this area is sensitive, and it can be irritated by the antiseptic. Antiseptic should be used only as advised by a doctor or nurse.

The other management steps that we use for lymphoedema of the leg, such as exercise, are not recommended for lymphoedema of the scrotum or penis, or for lymph scrotum.

Adjunct measures

Pubic hair. To help maintain good hygiene, and if culturally acceptable, men with genital swelling should keep the pubic hair short. Scissors should be used to cut the hair. Razors should never be used to shave the hair in this area, especially the scrotal sac.

Prophylactic antibiotics. Men with lymphoedema, elephantiasis, or lymph scrotum who continue to have recurrent acute attacks despite treatment with hygiene and medicated creams should be referred to a doctor or nurse for prophylactic antibiotics (Fig. 4.53, Chapter 4).

Preventing sexually transmitted diseases. Men with lymphoedema of the penis can use condoms to prevent sexually transmitted diseases and for birth control. Patients with lymphoedema of the penis should be referred to a doctor or nurse who can weigh the risks (condoms may make lymphoedema worse in some patients) and benefits (prevention of pregnancy and sexually transmitted disease).

Counselling. Feelings of embarrassment and shame, as well as sexual problems, are common among these men. Many of these patients do not participate in social activities and they avoid contact with other people. Some are able to hide their disease, but they need to know that they can keep their disease from getting worse. Counselling is often necessary for both the man and his partner. If sexual intercourse is still possible, advise the patient and his partner to wash their genital areas carefully both before and after intercourse. This may reduce the risk of acute attacks.

Surgery. Your patients with problems of the genital skin might ask you if their condition can be cured with surgery. For most of these men, hygiene and care of entry lesions are the only treatments available. A special type of surgery, known as "reconstructive" surgery, is now being developed for lymph scrotum and lymphoedema and elephantiasis of the scrotum and penis. This surgery is expensive, and it is not available in most places.

Severe oedema of the penis

In some patients, oedema of the penis can be so severe (Fig. 6.27) that it interferes with urination. If lymphoedema affects the foreskin, urine can be retained between the glans of the penis and the foreskin, causing additional problems. Severe lymphoedema makes it difficult to clean the penis, and this predisposes to bacterial infections and acute attacks.

Patients with advanced lymphoedema of the penis should be referred to a clinic where they can receive special attention and instruction, particularly on hygiene (Fig. 6.28). It may be necessary in some cases to massage the penis in order to temporarily decrease the lymphoedema and facilitate hygiene and urination (Fig. 6.29). Skilled health personnel, such as a nurse or a physician, can teach the patient how to do this without harming himself.

Acute attacks in the scrotum and penis

The symptoms of an acute attack in the scrotal area (Fig 6.30) are similar to those in the arms and legs (fever, headache, pain, and increased swelling, temperature, and redness in the affected area). A lump or swollen gland (lymph node) in the groin area may be the first sign immediately before an acute attack. Bacteria cause these acute attacks.

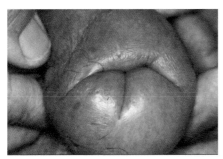

Fig. 6.27 Severe lymphoedema of the penis. It will be difficult for this patient to properly wash inside the fore-skin of the penis. He should be referred to a doctor, nurse, or clinic for further care and instruction.

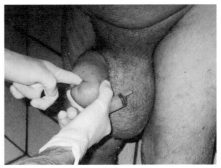

Fig. 6.28 Hygiene of the area inside the foreskin in severe lymphoedema of the penis. A physician is teaching the patient how to wash this area properly. The patient will need help with washing until his condition improves.

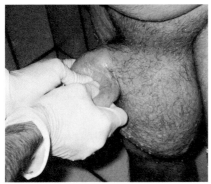

Fig. 6.29 Massage for lymphoedema of the penis. In a clinic, the physician is teaching the health worker and the patient how to massage the penis to reduce swelling and allow for proper washing. With experience, it will be possible for the patient to do massage and hygiene properly in his own home.

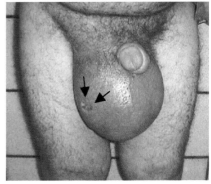

Fig. 6.30 Acute bacterial attack in the scrotum. The skin of the scrotum is tense, swollen, red, and very painful. A small entry lesion is visible on the right (arrows).

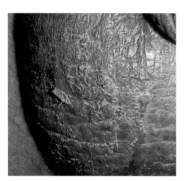

Fig. 6.31 Skin of the scrotum peeling after an acute attack. Peeling of the skin is also observed after acute attacks in the legs and arms.

After an acute attack, the skin of the scrotum or penis may peel (Fig 6.31), or become darker in colour (hyperpigmented).

Acute attack management

Acute attacks in the genital area (Fig. 6.30) require the same management as acute attacks in the limbs or breast, including referral to a doctor or nurse for certain patients.

- Use clean cold compresses to reduce pain and keep the area cool until the pain goes away.
- Tell your patients to take medicine to control their fever.
- If your patients develop blisters on the skin, tell them not to break them open, because more bacteria can enter the skin.
- As soon as your patients are able, once the pain subsides, they should continue with good hygiene, paying special attention to finding and treating entry lesions.
- Oral or injectable antibiotics are recommended for all of these patients— if they have the opportunity to be seen by the medical staff in the clinic, the drug is available, and the patient can afford it. Antibiotics can shorten the length of the attack, reduce the amount of additional lymphatic damage caused by the attack, and improve the patient's long-term prognosis.

With good hygiene, even though improvement may be slow, men with lymph scrotum or lymphoedema of the scrotum or penis can decrease the frequency of the acute attacks. You can tell your patients that good hygiene will prevent the disease from getting worse.

Important: If a patient develops increased volume of the scrotum with sudden, very severe pain in the testis (especially if he is young and has a normal-appearing scrotum and penis), he needs to be referred to a clinic for further evaluation as soon as possible. He may have testicular torsion, in which the blood vessels to the testis become twisted and the blood supply cut off, or he may have a bacterial infection inside the scrotal sac. He needs immediate medical attention.

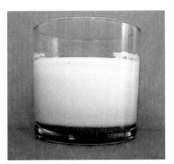

Fig. 6.32 Milky urine in a patient with chyluria, after eating a fatty meal.

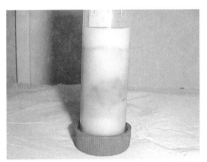

Fig. 6.33 Hemato-chyluria, in which the lymph fluid in the urine is mixed with blood. Patients may have various amounts of blood in the urine, resulting in urine ranging in colour from light pink to bloody red.

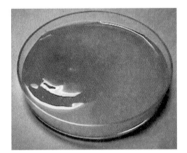

Fig. 6.34 Typical clot in the urine of a patient with chyluria. Clots vary in colour, depending on how much blood is present. Clots may be formed inside the bladder, which make it difficult to urinate (pee).

Urinary Tract Problems

In areas with lymphatic filariasis, people can have problems with their urine. These include:

• haematuria (red urine)
• chyluria (urine that is milky)

Haematuria

Haematuria is blood in the urine. Filariasis can cause haematuria, but many other diseases can also, including some that are very serious. As a health care worker in the community, you cannot directly help these patients without additional advice. So, if patients complain of red urine, you must refer them to a doctor or clinic.

Chyluria

Chyluria, or milky urine, can occur in men, women, and older children (usually older than 15 years). The white colour is caused by fats, which are found in many foods. From time to time the urine appears white, like milk (Fig. 6.32). If blood is also present, the urine may appear milky, mixed with a pink or red colour (Fig. 6.33).

Patients with chyluria, especially men, have trouble urinating (peeing). This problem occurs when a clot forms. These clots are passed in the urine. They vary in size and colour (Fig. 6.34). Chyluria also causes patients to lose weight and feel tired. If your patients have these problems often, they should see a doctor or nurse to be evaluated. Chyluria does not cause fever. If your patients have fever, you should refer them to a doctor for additional evaluation and care.

Men with chyluria may also have hydrocoele, lymph scrotum, or lymphoedema of the scrotum.

Management of chyluria

Chyluria is a very difficult condition to cure, but there is hope for people with chyluria! Chyluria can be managed by:

- eating foods that are low in fat and high in protein
- drinking lots of fluids
- resting during the episodes of milky urine
- not lifting heavy objects
- not walking up stairs during the episodes of milky urine.

You should talk with your patients and their families to explain the new diet. Fruits, vegetables, low fat meats, white meat, egg whites, and beans are foods that are low in fat and high in protein. Encourage your patients to share recipes and secrets of preparing good-tasting food made without fat.

Fatty foods should be avoided. These include, among others:

- any fried foods (Fig. 6.35)
- chocolate
- coconut
- avocado
- pork
- the skin and dark meat of chicken
- cheese and milk, especially goat milk
- the yellow part of eggs (yolk)
- oil, margarine, or butter (even to cook food).

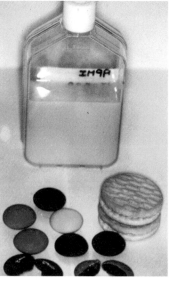

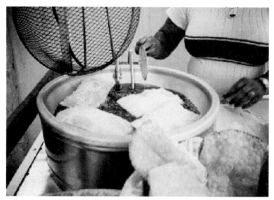

Fig. 6.35 Chyluria patients should avoid all kinds of fried foods.

Fig. 6.36 Even when your patient has adopted the right diet at home, if they eat "junk food", which contains hidden fat, the milky urine (shown in the bottle) can persist. Examples of junk food are shown.

Tips for management of chyluria
- Low-fat food is good for all family members, but young children should also eat foods that contain fat.
- Let your patients know that if they eat the wrong kinds of foods, the milky urine will reappear or get worse.
- Your patients need to see a doctor if the milky urine continues for more than 30 days, or reappears one or more times a month, even when they eat the recommended foods.

Alert: Be sure that your patients are not eating "hidden" fat which is present in many commercially prepared foods, especially so-called "junk food" (Fig. 6.36)

A nurse or nutritionist at the clinic or hospital can advise you about the best and most affordable local foods for your patients. A nutritionist may be able to advise you about the local availability of foods that contain a certain type of fat known as medium-chain triglycerides. This is the only type of fat that can be recommended for patients with chyluria.

Recommended Reading

Acton WH, Rao SS. The causation of lymph-scrotum. *Indian Med Gazette* 1930; 65:541–546.

Addiss DG, Dimock KA, Eberhard ML, Lammie PJ. Clinical, parasitologic and immunologic observations of patients with hydrocele and elephantiasis in an area with endemic lymphatic filariasis. *J Infect Dis* 1995; 171:755–758.

Addiss DG, Dreyer G. Treatment of Lymphatic Filariasis. In: Nutman TB, ed. *Lymphatic Filariasis.* London: Imperial College Press. 2000; 151–199

Dalela D, Kumar A, Ahlawat R, Goel TC, Mishra VK, Chandra H. Routine radio-imaging in filarial chyluria—is it necessary in developing countries? *Br J Urol* 1992; 69:291–293.

Diamond E, Schapira HE. Chyluria—a review of the literature. *Urology* 1985; 26:427–431.

Doi SQ, Meinertz H, Nilausen K, Faria EC, Quintao EC. Intestinal cholesterol absorption in the chyluria model. *J Lipid Res* 1987; 28:1129–36.

Dreyer G, Norões J, Addiss D. The silent burden of sexual disability associated with lymphatic filariasis. *Acta Tropica* 1997; 63:57–60

Dreyer G, Ottesen EA, Galdino E, Andrade L, Rocha A, Medeiros Z, Moura I, Cassimiro MI, Beliz MF, Coutinho A. Renal abnormalities in microfilaremic patients with bancroftian filariasis. *Am J Trop Med Hyg* 1992; 46:745–751.

Edwards BD, Eastwood JB, Shearer RJ. Chyluria as a cause of haematuria in patients from endemic areas. *Br J Urol* 1988; 62:609–611.

Gratama S. The pathogenesis of hydrocele in filarial infection. *Trop Geogr Med* 1969; 21:254–268.

Gyapong JO, Adjei S, Gyapong M, Asamoah G. Rapid community diagnosis of lymphatic filariasis. *Acta Tropica*; 1996; 61:65–74.

Gyapong JO, Webber RH, Morris J, Bennet S. Prevalence of hydrocele as a rapid diagnostic index for lymphatic filariasis. *Trans Roy Soc Trop Med Hyg* 1998; 92:40–43.

Hsieh JT, Chang HC, Law HS, Shun CT. Cyst-like chylous coagulum in the urinary bladder of a patient with recurrent chyluria. *J Formos Med Assoc* 1999; 98:586–588.

Norões J, Addiss D, Amaral F, Coutinho A, Medeiros Z, Dreyer G. Occurrence of adult *Wuchereria bancrofti* in the scrotal area of men with microfilaremia. *Trans Roy Soc Trop Med Hyg* 1996; 90:55–56.

Norões J, Addiss D, Santos A, Medeiros Z, Coutinho A, Dreyer G. Ultrasonographic evidence of abnormal lymphatic vessels in young men with adult *Wuchereria bancrofti* infection in the scrotal area. *J Urology* 1996; 156:409–412.

Ohyama C, Saita H, Miyasato N. Spontaneous remission of chyluria. *J Urol* 1979; 121:316–317.

Pettit J, Sawczuk IS. Use of lymphoscintigraphy in chyluria. *Urology* 1988; 32:367–369.

Quintao EC, Drewiacki A, Stechhaln K, de Faria EC, Sipahi AM. Origin of cholesterol transported in intestinal lymph: studies in patients with filarial chyluria. *J Lipid Res* 1979; 20:941–5.

Roosen JU, Larsen T, Iversen E, Berg JBS. A comparison of aspiration, antazoline sclerotherapy and surgery in the treatment of hydrocele. *Br J Urol* 1991; 68:404–406

Sherman RH, Goldman LB, deVere White RW. Filarial chyluria as a cause of acute urinary retention. *Urology* 1987; 29:642–645.

Warter J, Metais P, Berthier G, Bach A. Treatment of chyluria with a medium-chain triglyceride diet. *Pathol Biol* (Paris). 1972; 20:865–869.

Recommended Viewing

Lymphatic Filariasis: Hope for a better life. (Training video). Program for health care workers, 58 minutes.

For further information on the scientific publications please contact a university or medical school library, or write to Centers for Disease Control and Prevention (contact information on page 111).

Copies of the video may be purchased through the Public Health Foundation in the United States (contact information on page 111).

CHAPTER SEVEN

Factors That Complicate Lymphoedema Management in Filariasis-Endemic Areas

Persons living in tropical countries where lymphatic filariasis is endemic are exposed to other diseases that can complicate the management of their lymphoedema. In most cases, the principles of lymphoedema management proposed in this book will benefit these patients, but in some cases, lymphoedema management will need to be modified or complemented, and it may be incompatible with treatment for these other conditions. In this chapter, we briefly discuss some of these medical problems and suggest ways to address them.

Diseases of the Veins: Venous Insufficiency and Venous Ulcer

Venous ulcers (Fig 7.01) are caused by chronic venous insufficiency, or a lack of capacity of the veins of the lower limbs to return adequate amounts of blood to the heart. The veins become twisted, large, and tortuous, and are known as varices, or varicose veins. Venous ulcers are the most common form of leg ulcers, both in filariasis-endemic and non-endemic areas. As with lymphoedema, venous disease has a significant negative impact on quality of life and ability to work. Women tend to be more prone to develop venous disease than men, and obesity increases this risk. As with lymphoedema of the leg, the prevalence of venous ulcers increases with increasing age, although some patients develop them before 30 years of age.

Most venous ulcers are located above the ankle near the medial malleolus (Fig. 7.02), the remainder being located elsewhere on the leg or foot. Either or both legs can be affected. Venous ulcers may be single or multiple; if left untreated, the ulcer can involve the entire circumference of the leg (Fig. 7.03).

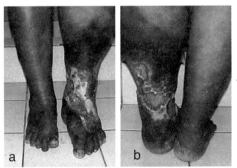

Fig. 7.01 Venous ulcer in a patient with lymphoedema. Front (a) and back (b) views. Note the hyperpigmentation of the surrounding skin, which is very common in this disease.

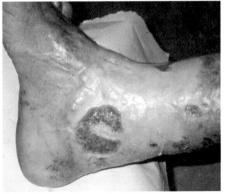

Fig. 7.02 Venous ulcer in a typical location – near the medial malleolus. This ulcer is in the process of healing; note the lighter colour and thinness (atrophy) of the skin around the ulcer.

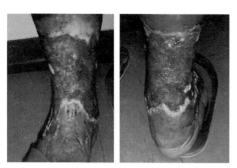

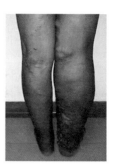

Fig. 7.03 Venous ulcer involving the entire circumference of the leg.

Fig. 7.04 Lymphoedema and venous insufficiency. This patient has worse venous insufficiency in the right leg, as well as lymphoedema. Note the large varices above the knees.

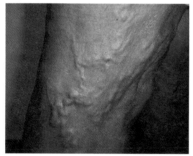

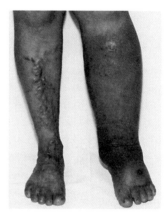

Fig. 7.05 Venous varices. The veins protrude and are dilated and twisted (tortuous).

Fig. 7.06 A patient with bilateral venous insufficiency and lymphoedema of the left leg. It is much easier to see the varicose veins in the right leg , which has no lymphoedema. The degree of venous insufficiency was similar in both legs, as measured in a special examination known as ultrasonography with Doppler.

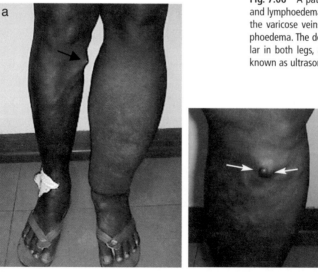

Fig. 7.07 A patient with a varicose button on the right leg (Fig 7.07 a, arrow). The patient has venous insufficiency of the left leg, but it cannot be seen easily because she also has lymphoedema of the left leg. She also has a venous ulcer on the lower right leg (gauze). Fig 7.07 b is a close-up view of the varicose button (arrows).

Patients with lymphoedema frequently have varying degrees of venous insufficiency as well (Fig. 7.04 and 7.05). However, it may be difficult to see twisted, enlarged varices in patients who have lymphoedema (Fig. 7.06). As the leg decreases in size with lymphoedema management, the varices are more easily seen. Patients with venous varices may also have a "varicose button"—a dilated section of vein very close to the surface of the skin (Fig. 7.07), which bleeds easily if traumatized. Bleeding can be severe enough to require medical attention.

Venous ulcers produce pain and discomfort, which do not correlate well with the size of the ulcer. Most painful are the deep ulcers, particularly those near the malleolus, or small venous ulcers surrounded by whitish skin. Patients commonly complain of swelling and aching of the legs, often worse at the end of the day, which improves with leg elevation. Those with severe pain may have a secondary infection, or another, non-venous, cause for the ulcer. Venous ulcers have a peculiar odour and often drain fluid. Itching of the surrounding skin is also common. Recurrence of the ulcer at the same site is characteristic of venous ulcer disease.

In addition to ulcers, venous insufficiency produces a variety of skin changes. Hyperpigmentation (Fig 7.01), often reddish-brown in colour, is common, as is eczema, characterized by redness, scaling, itching, and occasionally exudates. This eczema is known as venous dermatitis. It is often made worse by topical medications, which cause allergic reactions in these patients.

The management of venous ulcers is more complicated than that of lymphoedema, although in principle the basic components of lymphoedema management will not harm patients with venous ulcers. These patients should be referred to a clinic. Hygiene and care of entry lesions between the toes are particularly important in persons with venous insufficiency. Topical medications in the ulcers should be avoided, unless prescribed by a doctor or nurse. Rest and elevation of the leg are essential in venous insufficiency. Elevation above the level of the heart for 30 minutes 3 to 4 times per day is recommended. In advanced venous disease, elevation may not be sufficient. Compressive measures are the cornerstone of therapy for patients with venous ulcer (Fig. 7.08).

Diabetes (High Levels of Blood Sugar)

Patients with diabetes have many medical problems. For health workers in filariasis-endemic areas, the effects of diabetes on the skin are particularly important. Ulcers occur on the legs and feet, and gangrene may develop. In severe cases, the leg must be amputated; more commonly, amputation is limited to the toes. Delayed wound healing and increased risk of infection are very common in people with diabetes. For your patients with lymphoedema who also have diabetes and entry lesions between the toes, hygiene alone is unlikely to clear the entry lesions. Rather than waiting to see if hygiene alone will clear these lesions, antifungal cream is recommended right away, regardless of the stage of lymphoedema. These entry lesions usually are more

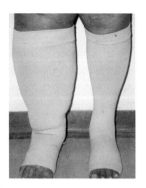

Fig. 7.08 Compression. Compressive measures, such as special bandages and specially-fitted stockings, can be very helpful for your patients with venous insufficiency and lymphoedema. This patient has been fitted with compressive stockings, which are usually expensive and should be prescribed by a doctor or therapist if the patient can afford them.

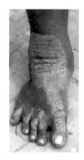

Fig. 7.09 Psoriasis. This patient has typical silver, scaly lesions on the foot and lower leg.

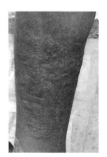

Fig. 7.10 Active psoriasis. Patients with psoriasis have acute inflammatory reactions, which should not be confused with an acute bacterial attack in a patient with lymphoedema. This is the same patient shown in Fig 7.09.

"resistant" to antifungal treatment than are those in people who do not have diabetes.

Psoriasis

Psoriasis (Fig. 7.09) is a chronic disease of the skin that waxes and wanes in intensity. It tends to cluster in families. The skin lesions are distinctive and have four prominent features: the margins of the lesion have clear-cut borders; the surface of the lesion is covered with silvery scales; the skin underneath the scale is uniform, glossy, and pinkish in colour; and small droplets of blood appear on the skin within a few seconds after the scales are scraped off.

Patients with psoriasis complain about the unsightly appearance of the lesions, which may cause low self-esteem and social isolation. The lesions itch and are sometimes painful, especially when the palms of the hands, soles of the feet, or spaces between the toes and fingers are involved.

Health workers in filariasis-endemic areas should be aware that:

- Treatment of psoriasis can be difficult; patients with psoriasis should be referred to a clinic for further evaluation and specific treatment.
- The scaling lesions should not be confused with the peeling of the skin that occurs after acute attacks (Fig. 5.03).
- The scales of psoriasis should not be removed with hygiene.
- The red plaque-like lesions of active psoriasis can be confused with an acute attack (Fig. 7.10); unlike acute attacks, these lesions are not associated with high fever and the other systemic signs and symptoms described in Chapter 5.

Leprosy

Patients with leprosy may have knobs on the skin that can be confused with those of the lymphoedema related to lymphatic filariasis. Leprosy patients often have skin lesions that are hypopigmented and reddish in colour, and there is a loss of sensation at the site. This loss of sensitivity leads to destruction of the toes, as well as ulcers, especially on the bottom (plantar surface) of the foot. Patients with unusual knobs or skin lesions should be referred to a clinic for further evaluation.

Myiasis

Human myiasis occurs when fly (*Diptera*) larvae or maggots infest human tissues. Primary myiasis occurs when the larvae themselves cause the break in the skin. In secondary myiasis, the female fly lays her eggs in or near an entry lesion or wound, and the larvae (maggots) develop and enter the wound (Fig. 7.11). Maggots may remain superficial or penetrate to the deep tissues. Myiasis in the subcutaneous tissues (furuncular myiasis) can be mistaken for an abscess.

The mainstay of treatment for myiasis is extraction of the larvae. No substances should be put onto the wound in an attempt to kill the larvae. Severe forms of myiasis may require incision under local anaesthesia to extract the larvae. For furuncular myiasis only, a form of myiasis found in Africa, petroleum jelly can be applied to suffocate the maggots.

Myiasis can complicate the management of lymphoedema, particularly in patients with advanced elephantiasis.

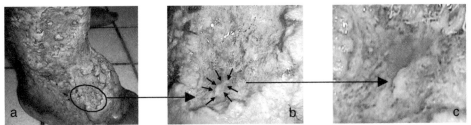

Fig. 7.11   Myiasis in a patient with lymphoedema and a venous ulcer (a). Myiasis results from flies laying their eggs in damaged tissue. Figures 7.11 b and c show a close-up view of the larvae (arrows).

Pregnancy

Many pregnant women develop swelling of the legs, which is usually caused by venous insufficiency. This venous insufficiency, in turn, can lead to a secondary lymphoedema. Thus, women with lymphoedema in filariasis-endemic areas frequently report its onset during pregnancy. The venous insufficiency of pregnancy may also cause worsening of pre-existing lymphoedema. In both these situations, the basic components of lymphoedema management should be followed. Compression may become more important as an adjunct measure during pregnancy. Other medical problems, including malnutrition and pre-eclampsia, may also contribute to worsening of oedema in pregnancy. Any pregnant woman with severe oedema, but especially those with symmetrical oedema, should be referred to a clinic for further evaluation.

After delivery, even if the lymphoedema of pregnancy decreases or disappears, hygiene and other measures should be continued. These measures will help prevent acute attacks and help avoid recurrence of the lymphoedema. After delivery, daily hygiene should be used for the breast (before and after breast-feeding) and the armpits.

Occlusive and Semi-occlusive Dressings

Occlusion of the skin (by surrounding it with an impermeable material, such as a plastic dressing or other material) and semi-occlusion of the skin (with a semi-permeable material) have profound effects that can produce, aggravate, or be used to treat a variety of skin diseases. Occlusion and semi-occlusion are used to treat psoriasis, to prevent myiasis, and to treat venous ulcer wounds that are draining or leaking, for example. However, they can also increase the growth of skin bacteria and lead to fungal infections, which, in people with lymphoedema, provide entry lesions for bacteria and opportunities for acute attacks.

A wide range of materials for occlusive dressings is commercially available in developed countries. For patients in filariasis-endemic countries who need occlusive dressings, the choices are more restricted, as these materials tend to be expensive. Lymphoedema patients with psoriasis, myiasis, or wounds that continue to drain fluid may benefit from occlusive or semi-occlusive dressings. These patients should be referred to a clinic for further evaluation and treatment.

Recommended Reading

Freedberg IM, Eisen AZ, Wolff K, Austen KF, Goldsmith LA, Katz SI, Fitzpatrick TB, eds. *Fitzpatrick's Dermatology in General Medicine* 1999; McGraw-Hill, New York.

Morison M, Moffatt C, Bridel-Nixon J, Bale S, eds. *Nursing Management of Chronic Wounds.* second edition, 1997; Mosby, London.

Valencia IC, Falabella A, Kirsner RS, Eaglstein WH. Chronic venous insufficiency and venous leg ulceration. *J Am Acad Dermatology* 2001; 44:401–21.

Wirtz RA, Azad AF. Myiasis. In: Strickland, GT, ed. *Hunter's Tropical Medicine and Emerging Infectious Diseases—8th ed.* 2000; 916–918, WB Saunders, Philadelphia.

For further information on the scientific publications please contact a university or medical school library, or write to Centers for Disease Control and Prevention (contact information on page 111).

CHAPTER EIGHT
Differential Diagnosis

People living in tropical countries where lymphatic filariasis is endemic are exposed to many other diseases that also can cause swelling or disfiguration of the legs, arms, breast, and genitals. It can be difficult in many cases to distinguish these from lymphatic filariasis; there is no laboratory test that can determine with absolute certainty that lymphatic filariasis alone is the cause of lymphoedema, hydrocoele, or other clinical manifestations.

In many cases, the management of these conditions is the same, regardless of the original cause of lymphatic damage. In other cases, the treatment may differ and the correct diagnosis is important. As you gain experience with lymphoedema management, you will become familiar with the clinical manifestations related to lymphatic filariasis and you will become more certain about which patients to refer to a clinic or hospital for further evaluation. In this chapter, we offer a few tips on some of these other conditions that can be confused with manifestations of lymphatic filariasis.

Swelling of Limbs

Chronic lymphoedema associated with lymphatic filariasis is triggered by one or more acute bacterial attacks. Pay special attention to patients whose lymphoedema begins without such an attack (this is known as "cold lymphoedema"). These patients may have been born with defective lymphatic vessels (i.e., congenital abnormalities), or may have other causes of lymphoedema. This is especially true when the onset of lymphoedema occurs during childhood (especially before puberty) or after the age of 40 years. These patients should be evaluated by a doctor or nurse.

In filariasis-endemic areas, lymphoedema of the arms is much less common than lymphoedema of the legs. Surgical removal of the axillary lymph nodes, whether with mastectomy (for treatment of breast cancer) or with other medical procedures, is an important cause of lymphoedema of the upper limbs (Fig. 8.01), both in filariasis-endemic and non-endemic countries. Patients with lymphoedema of the arm, whether due to congenital abnormalities or to other causes, will benefit from the principles of lymphoedema management proposed in this book, but they should also be monitored by a doctor or nurse.

Pay special attention to children with lymphoedema. Lymphatic filariasis does not cause lymphoedema in young children, regardless of whether it is accompanied by skin changes characteristic of lymphoedema in filariasis-endemic areas (such as knobs, vesicles, or wart-like lesions). Thus, children with lymphoedema (Fig. 8.02,

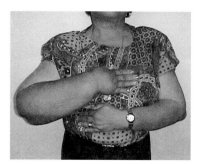

Fig. 8.01 Lymphoedema of the right arm after mastectomy with removal of axillary lymph nodes, not related to filarial disease.

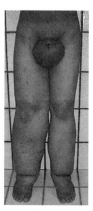

Fig. 8.02 Congenital lymphoedema in a 14 year-old boy, which affects the lower limbs, buttocks, penis, and scrotal sac. The swelling began immediately after he was born.

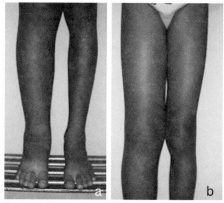

Fig. 8.03 a, b A 10 year-old boy who developed a "cold lymphoedema" of the right leg when he was 8 years old. The lymphoedema affects the thigh as well (b). The penis and scrotal sac are normal (not shown).

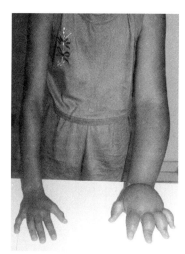

Fig. 8.04 Congenital swelling. A 13 year-old girl who was born with swelling of the left arm due to a benign soft tissue tumour, which was misdiagnosed as lymphoedema.

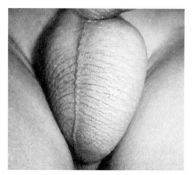

Fig. 8.05 Left hydrocoele in a 3 year-old boy, not related to lymphatic filariasis.

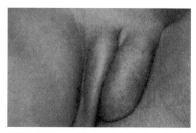

Fig. 8.06 Oedema of the genitals (labia majora), worse on the left, in an 8 year-old girl. The oedema was caused by a mass in the abdomen, not by lymphatic filariasis

8.03) or any kind of swelling (Fig. 8.04) should be evaluated by a doctor or nurse promptly to determine the underlying cause.

Swelling of the Genitals and Breast

Lymphatic filariasis does not cause hydrocoele in young children (Fig. 8.05). Swelling of the genitals (Fig. 8.06) in a female of any age, or swelling of the breast in children (Fig. 8.07) are rarely, if ever, caused by lymphatic filariasis. Other causes, including tumours and congenital abnormalities, are much more likely.

Lipedema

Lipedema is a chronic swelling disease caused by excess fatty tissue, usually in the upper legs, thighs, and hips. Both sides are usually involved. The hands and feet are usually normal. In most cases, lipedema develops during puberty or 1 to 2 years later. Some patients with lipedema also have lymphatic vessel lesions, and they develop a condition called lipo-lymphoedema (Fig 8.08). Once chronic lymphoedema becomes established, the patients are more susceptible to acute attacks and to develop entry lesions. Thus, patients with lipedema will generally benefit from the basic lymphoedema management techniques proposed in this book.

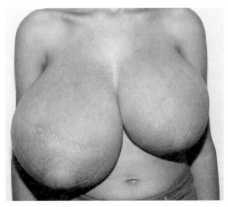

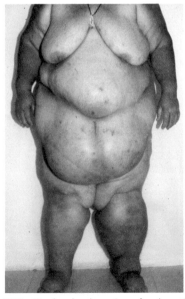

Fig. 8.07 A 10 year-old girl with a massive increase in breast volume, six months after its onset. This was not related to filariasis.

Fig. 8.08 Lipo-lymphoedema in a female patient. Note the lymphoedema in both lower limbs (greater in the left leg). Skin lesions were found in all the interdigital spaces and the patient had already had several bacterial acute attacks.

Knobs

The frequency and pattern of knobs associated with lymphatic filariasis vary from country to country. These patterns relate to cultural practices, such as cutting the skin as a traditional treatment for lymphoedema, biological factors, such as production of keloid tissue at the site of a scar, and other factors.

- Knobs are also caused by other diseases, and you should be alert to the possibility that unusual-appearing knobs may not be caused by lymphoedema related to lymphatic filariasis. These patients should be referred to a physician or nurse for further evaluation.

- Knobs with rapid growth, with or without bleeding, must be due to other diseases like skin cancer.

- Mycetoma (Fig. 8.09) is a chronic localized infection caused by different species of fungi, which are found in the soil and on a variety of plants. The fungi gain access to the tissues during a penetrating injury. Abscesses develop, which contain clusters of the fungi, known as "grains". The abscesses may communicate to the surface of the skin through sinuses, or may involve nearby bone. The lesions cause local swelling, and may be quite painful just before the sinus tracts emerge onto the skin surface. These patients will not benefit from the lymphoedema management proposed in this book. They should be referred to a clinic for special treatment. In advanced cases, surgery, usually amputation, is done, but, as mycetoma is not a life-threatening illness, this is not often recommended for less-advanced cases.

- Chromoblastomycosis is a chronic fungal infection of the skin and subcutaneous tissues caused by pigmented fungi that can be found on wood, on plant debris, or in soil. Infection follows injuries involving the feet, legs, arms (Fig. 8.10), or upper trunk. The lesions often become secondarily infected with bacteria. Complications of chromoblastomycosis include local lymphoedema and elephantiasis, as well as certain types of skin tumours. It is important to differentiate chromoblastomycosis from mossy lesions.

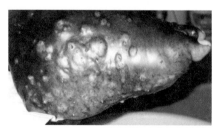

Fig. 8.09 Knobs on the foot of a patient with mycetoma, a disease caused by infection with a specific type of fungi.

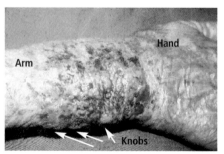

Fig. 8.10 Knobs on the arm of a patient with chromoblastomycosis, a disease caused by infection with a specific type of fungi (courtesy of Dr. Valdir Bandeira).

Milky Urine

In bancroftian filariasis-endemic areas, lymphatic filariasis causes the vast majority of cases of milky, fatty urine, or chyluria. However, chyluria can also be caused by lymphatic malformations, pregnancy, trauma, tumours, surgery, or other parasitic diseases. Regardless of the underlying cause of chyluria, all of these patients will benefit from a low-fat high-protein diet. In a child, chyluria is unlikely to be due to filariasis. Prompt referral is required for further evaluation.

Other conditions may mimic chyluria. For example, patients with diabetes can have "milky urine" caused by pus. Thus, patients with diabetes who develop "milky urine" should be sent to the hospital for evaluation, even if they do not have fever. To distinguish between these two conditions, ask the patient to urinate into a transparent container and let the urine sit for approximately 30–40 minutes. If a clear separation develops between what appears to be normal urine and a layer of sediment in the bottom of the container, the patient does not have chyluria.

Inguinal Hernia

Inguinal hernia, or the protrusion of a loop of intestine through an abnormal opening between the abdomen and the scrotal sac, may mimic hydrocoele. Usually, the "base" (or top) of a hydrocoele is narrow when the patient stands (Fig. 8.11). In contrast, with a hernia, the base is normally wide (Fig. 8.12). In either case the patient should be seen by a physician.

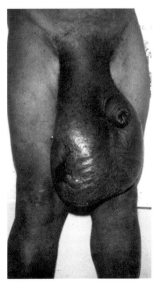

Fig. 8.11 A man with a large hydrocoele. The base (top) of most hydrocoeles is narrow, while in hernia it is much wider. Note in this patient how far the penis is from the base of the hydrocoele.

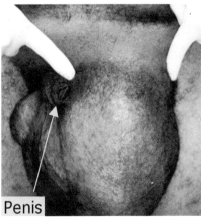

Penis

Fig. 8.12 Inguinal hernia. Note how wide the base of the hernia is, compared with hydrocoele. Unilateral hernia can be easily distinguished from lymphoedema of the scrotal sac, which involves the whole sac.

Recommended Reading

Hay RJ. Chromoblastomycosis. In: Strickland, GT, ed. *Hunter's Tropical Medicine and Emerging Infectious Diseases – 8th ed.* 2000; 542–544, WB Saunders, Philadelphia.

Hay RJ. Mycetoma. In: Strickland, GT, ed. *Hunter's Tropical Medicine and Emerging Infectious Diseases – 8th ed.* 2000; 537–541, WB Saunders, Philadelphia.

Meyers WM. Leprosy. In: Strickland, GT, ed. *Hunter's Tropical Medicine and Emerging Infectious Diseases – 8th ed.* 2000; 513–523, WB Saunders, Philadelphia.

Weissleder H, Schuchhardt C, eds. *Lymphoedema Diagnosis and Therapy.* 1997; Kagerer Kommunikation, Bonn.

For further information on the scientific publications please contact a university or medical school library, or write to Centers for Disease Control and Prevention (contact information on page 111).

CHAPTER NINE
Achieving, Maintaining, and Monitoring Lymphoedema Programs

In this chapter we would like to share a few observations and suggestions based on our experience of working with patients in Recife, Brazil and Leogane, Haiti, and on discussions with colleagues in Africa, India, and China. Our hope is that this experience will be helpful to others who are interested in developing lymphoedema management programs in other filariasis-endemic areas.

Achieving Success

Lymphatic filariasis and the people who suffer its chronic consequences have long been neglected. For years, both physicians and patients have been told that elephantiasis is the "end stage of filarial disease", and that little could be done to prevent its progression. Thus, one of the most challenging barriers to successful lymphoedema treatment is a lack of hope—a fatalistic belief that progression of the disease is inevitable. This belief is common among patients and health workers alike in filariasis-endemic areas. When combined with the social isolation that people with lymphoedema often suffer, this fatalism leads to dependency, passivity, and despondency.

At the same time, patients may be reluctant to believe that the simple measures presented in this book will be of much help to them. They may be looking for a dramatic, instant cure, a strong medicine that can quickly reverse the underlying lymphatic damage. They may become impatient with the daily discipline required to practice the techniques described in this book.

Thus, as a health worker, providing realistic hope is one of the most important things you can do for lymphoedema patients.

To realize this hope, your patients must learn new ideas, develop new skills, and become motivated to practice these new management techniques.

- Your educational messages must be culturally appropriate and readily understandable by the patients.
- *Patients are responsible for their own care.* As a health care worker, your job is to empower your patients with new knowledge, new skills, and new motivation. Except for patients with very advanced disease (stage 7) who require continual monitoring and care from the health system, your job is not to "do for" the patients, but to empower them (and their families) to "do for" themselves. Sometimes, after learning the techniques described in this book, health workers may be hesitant to fully share their new expertise. Perhaps they fear that if they share this knowledge with their patients, their expertise will no longer be needed and their job will be threatened. Or perhaps they think that patients

will improve more if the health worker, a "trained professional" takes care of the daily hygiene and skin care. Nothing could be farther from the truth! Such an attitude is harmful because it unnecessarily creates dependency on the health worker and decreases patient motivation. The role of the health worker, the clinic, and the hospital is to support the patient in her or his daily lymphoedema self-care, which, except in unusual circumstances, is best done at home or in the community.

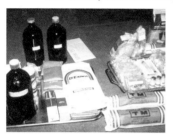

Fig. 9.01 A tray of options for lymphoedema care. Soap, medicated creams, antiseptic solution, antibiotics, and bandages are available. The patient can benefit from some or all of these items.

Lymphoedema care is life-long. To be successful, the patient must be able to practice the basic principles described in this book on a daily basis. As a health worker, you can provide your patients with accurate information about lymphoedema, teach them the skills they need to care for themselves, and provide them ongoing support and motivation. In this way, you offer your patients a "tray of opportunity" (Fig. 9.01). With your guidance, patients can master the basic principles of lymphoedema self-care. In addition, your patients can select "optional items" from the tray of lymphoedema care (for example, bandages) if they can afford them and can use them properly.

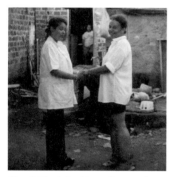

Fig. 9.02 A health worker can learn from patients as well as teach them. Always ask your patient for their ideas, challenges, and concerns about their participation in the lymphoedema care programme.

- *Listen carefully to your patients and treat them with respect and compassion* (Fig. 9.02). Your patients can be your "teachers" for learning how best to help them. They can help you to find creative solutions to problems and challenges that arise in trying to adapt the principles in this book to their own realities.

- Family members, particularly children, should learn the principles of lymphoedema and be involved in the treatment process (Fig. 9.03). Family members can assist the patient with hygiene and skin care, particularly if the patient has advanced disease. They can also provide motivation and support.

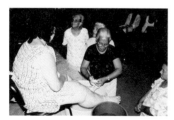

Fig. 9.03 Family members and friends should be involved in lymphoedema care. Here we see friends and neighbours learning how to do hygiene correctly. After learning, they will be prepared to help.

- Children are an important target group for lymphoedema education. In filariasis-endemic areas, many children have hidden damage caused by the filarial parasite. Good hygiene and skin care can prevent these children from developing lymphoedema (Fig. 9.04). In addition, educating children is an effective way to rapidly educate the entire community and reinforce the messages being taught to the patients. For these reasons, we can create *Hope Clubs for Kids* (see below).

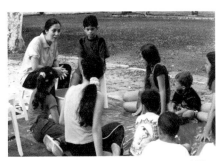

Fig. 9.04 Prevention is a great weapon. Children living in filariasis-endemic areas will benefit from practicing hygiene, which will prevent the first entry lesions and the development of acute attacks. In this way they can prevent lymphoedema. Here, a child is having his leg washed as an example for other children with no apparent disease.

Maintaining Success

Maintaining successful lymphoedema management depends on 1) finding creative solutions to challenges that arise; 2) periodically reinforcing the basic principles of lymphoedema care; and 3) sustaining patient motivation.

Listen to your patients and encourage them to help find solutions to problems that they encounter in trying to make lymphoedema care part of their daily routine. Patients themselves initially suggested many of the tips and techniques in this book.

Even patients who faithfully follow the steps of lymphoedema self-care will remain interested in a "cure" for their disease. Patients are influenced by the advice of their friends and neighbours, and by rumours of alternative treatments. Some of these other practices are harmless—these should not be discouraged if your patient finds comfort in them. Some may actually be helpful—these should be encouraged. However some are harmful, and these need to be discouraged. Examples of harmful practices include putting hot water on the skin during acute attacks, popping blisters, or cutting the skin (a practice known as scarification). We have found that patients usually need to be reminded of the basic principles of lymphoedema care at least once every 6 months. Otherwise, their knowledge and practices of lymphoedema care tend to drift, and they may begin to adopt ideas or practices that are potentially harmful.

Our experience in Brazil and Haiti during the last 5 to 10 years indicates that, if properly instructed and supported, patients remain motivated, and they continue their daily routine of hygiene, skin care, elevation, and exercises. One of the most effective and fun ways to maintain and reinforce patient motivation is to create *Hope Clubs*, in which patients support each other and prepare themselves once again for full participation as human beings and members of society.

Hope Clubs

Hope Clubs are the result of an innovative approach that was launched nine years ago in Recife, Brazil, at the Aggeu Magalhães Research Centre—FIOCRUZ. Currently the program is supported by the Federal University of Pernambuco and the Amaury Coutinho Non-Governmental Organization, created in December 1997. The aim of Hope Clubs is to give patients the skills, motivation, and enthusiasm to sustain effective, low-cost, and convenient self-care for their lymphoedema, and to amplify these activities throughout filariasis-endemic communities. Through group participation

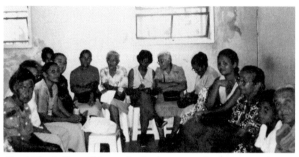

Fig. 9.05 A Hope Club meeting in the community. Patients gather to learn new skills, exchange life experiences, and propose solutions to new challenges

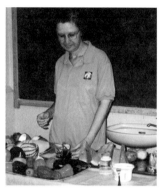

Fig. 9.06 A health worker is explaining to Chyluria Club members which kinds of foods are best for them and how to prepare good meals without fat.

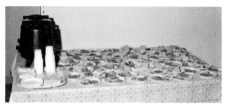

Fig. 9.07 Bon appétit! A new low-fat high protein recipe will be tested today. The food will be distributed among Chyluria Club members for their approval.

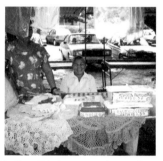

Fig. 9.08 Hope Fair. A moment where patients can display and sell their handcrafted work. The patients have a better life now. They can be healthier, more productive, and contribute to the financial support of the family.

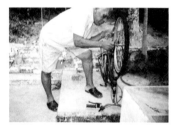

Fig. 9.09 Productive work. After learning how to prevent acute attacks of the scrotal sac, this patient is back to work.

and support, patients are encouraged to accept responsibility for the success or failure of their own management and to make the best use of their own resources (physical, emotional, social, and environmental) (Fig. 9.05). In Brazil, different Hope Clubs have been created for men and for women, and several Hope Clubs for Kids and Chyluria Clubs have also been established (9.06, 9.07).

Through participating in Hope Clubs, patients with lymphoedema come to realize that they are not alone; that they have access to simple, effective measures to prevent acute attacks and relieve suffering; that they can regain their potential for productive work (Figs. 9.08 and 9.09); that, as human beings, they have certain rights deserving recognition and respect; that, as social creatures, they and their family members can work together to help each other and to solve problems through cooperative action; and, that through such action, they can produce sustainable, positive changes within the community. For example, in Recife, where recent droughts have decreased access to clean water, Hope Club participants mobilized the community and established "foot-washing centres" where patients can gather and practice regular, daily hygiene. In other filariasis-endemic areas, people with lymphoedema have become volunteer leaders and advocates of mass treatment with antifilarial drugs to stop transmission of *W. bancrofti* in the community.

Addressing Challenges

Possible undesirable effects of a lymphoedema program

In Brazil, a few patients became so focused on their lymphoedema management and spent so much time on the self-care measures (such as elevating the leg virtually all the time and washing the leg many times each day), that it disrupted their own lives and the lives of their families. To avoid this, remind your patients that lymphoedema management is life-long, and that, although it is a powerful means to improve the quality of their lives, it is not an end in itself. Finding ways to integrate lymphoedema management into their daily activities can help your patients avoid making the strict practice of these measures their only priority.

Amputation: a solution or a problem?

Patients with advanced lymphoedema and their families may ask about amputation as a solution to their problem. The suffering that they experience is so great that they would prefer to live without the affected leg. In our experience, amputation is rarely a good option. Usually, the disease extends at least as high as the knee, so that an amputation below the knee, which has the best outcome, is not recommended. Even when the leg is amputated above the knee, lymphoedema tends to develop again at the site of the remaining stump.

Patients who insist on having an amputation should have a comprehensive medical and psychological evaluation to guarantee that there are no medical contraindications to the operation, that they have carefully considered the financial and other limitations of life without the leg, and that they are psychologically stable and consistent in their desire for amputation. After patients begin to participate in a lymphoedema care program, they start to feel better, their condition improves, they feel more hopeful, and they usually give up on the idea of amputation. As a health worker, it is important that you be available to patients who are considering amputation and their families to provide them with the knowledge and confidence they need to make the right decision while taking full advantage of lymphoedema treatment as described in this book.

If amputation is done, prevention of bacterial acute attacks is absolutely essential; all the tools available to prevent bacterial acute attacks, including prophylactic antibiotics, must be used for a long time. Thus, even after amputation, continual attention from the health care system is required.

Community Resources

Challenges to maintaining successful lymphoedema management programs include passivity and hopelessness among patients and their families, resulting from their long-standing beliefs that no effective treatment exists; lack of access to clean water; and lack of resources. Increasingly, potential donors are learning about the global effort to eliminate lymphatic filariasis, and they are expressing interest in helping to provide care for people with lymphoedema. These donors include non-governmental development organizations, religious groups, and manufacturers of medical supplies and skin care products (such as medicated creams). You may find that in your area, such groups are interested in helping support your lymphoedema management activities. We encourage you to talk with the leaders of these groups, and take advantage of opportunities to spread the word that, indeed, there is hope for people with lymphoedema in filariasis-endemic areas.

Benefits of Successful Lymphoedema Management

With good lymphoedema care, patients commonly experience short-term, medium-term and long-term benefits. In Recife, Brazil, patients typically realize these benefits within 2–3 weeks, 2–3 months, and up to 1 year, respectively. However, considerable variation occurs from patient to patient, and the rate at which individual patients experience the benefits of lymphoedema management depends on many factors, including cultural beliefs and practices, staff training, availability of clean water and supplies, and the patients' psychological, economic, and family situations.

Short-term benefits
- A decrease in bad odour
- Hope
- Motivation to fight the disease
- A sense of well-being and cleanliness after hygiene
- Self-acceptance
- Acceptance by the family

Intermediate-term benefits
- Decrease in frequency of acute attacks
- Disappearance of entry lesions (Fig. 9.10 a, b)
- Improvement of severe lesions, such as mossy foot (Fig. 9.11 a, b)
- Improved sense of well-being
- Improved self-esteem (as evidenced by a change in clothes, improved personal hygiene, care of hair and nails, and use of makeup in women)

Long-term benefits
- Increased independence

- Increased socialization
- Motivation to learn new ideas and skills
- Return to work
- Healthier sexual life
- Restoration of personal dignity

Monitoring Success

Improvement of the patient's condition increases motivation, which leads to further success. But how can this success best be measured? The following indicators may be useful.

SUGGESTED INDICATORS FOR MONITORING SUCCESS AT THE PATIENT LEVEL

Reduction and elimination of bad odour

Reduction in number and extent of entry lesions between the toes (fig. 9.10).

Frequency of acute attacks

Because of their strong link with disease progression and the pain and suffering that they cause, a decreased frequency of acute attacks is an important indicator for

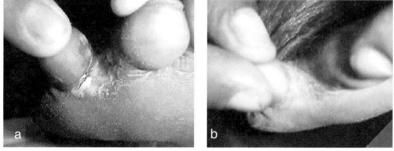

Fig. 9.10 An example of successful management of an entry lesion between the toes, before (a) and three weeks after beginning treatment (b). Medicated cream was necessary to cure this entry lesion.

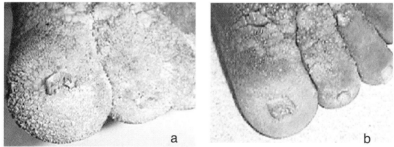

Fig. 9.11 Mossy lesions on the foot, before (a) and 6 months after beginning treatment (b). This patient was treated with medicated creams and systemic prophylactic antibiotics, as recommended for stage 6 lymphoedema. Note the improvement in the condition of the patient's toenails.

monitoring the success of lymphoedema management. Before and after starting treatment, patients can be asked the following questions:

- How many acute attacks did you have during the last year?
- How long has it been since the last acute attack?

Be careful not to blame your patients if they have an acute attack after beginning treatment. Instead, together with the patient, explore what factors might have contributed to the acute attack and encourage the patient to continue efforts to prevent acute attacks.

Skin condition
Proper, regular hygiene and skin care will improve the condition of the skin.

- If the skin is usually dirty, the patient is not washing correctly.
- With proper lymphoedema management, the number of entry lesions will decrease, and those that exist will be smaller.

Quality of life
Proper lymphoedema management improves quality of life. Standardized measures of quality of life have not yet been developed for persons with lymphoedema in filariasis-endemic areas. However, patients will often report improvements in a sense of well-being, self-confidence, and ability to work and participate in social activities (Fig. 9.12). You can monitor these changes through questions such as the following:

- What can you do now that you could not do last year?
- How do you feel about yourself?
- How are your family and friends treating you?

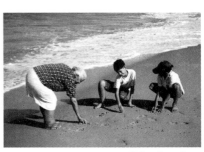

Fig. 9.12. Improving quality of life. After a long period of isolation, a grandmother's health and self-esteem have improved with the treatment of her lymphoedema. Now she can enjoy life with her grandsons.

OTHER INDICATORS OF PROGRAM SUCCESS

In addition to these individual indicators of success, you will want to keep track of a variety of *program* indicators, perhaps on a quarterly basis. These may include:

- Number of patients seen in the clinic, by lymphoedema stage
- Number of home visits to encourage patients and reinforce proper lymphoedema management
- Percentage of patients who can demonstrate proper lymphoedema management techniques
- Number of new patients referred by others
- Number of new patients participating in Hope Clubs

WHY NOT MONITOR LEG VOLUME AS AN INDICATOR OF SUCCESS?

During the early 1990s, recommendations were made to monitor leg volume using a "water-displacement" method, in which patients put their leg into a tub full of water, and the water that flowed out of the tub was measured. This method was time-consuming, messy, and used lots of water. In addition, some patients had dramatic changes in leg volume, while others did not, even though they faithfully followed all the steps of lymphoedema management. Focusing on volume reduction as the main indicator of success was discouraging for these patients. Even more significantly, volume reduction did not seem to correlate well with other indicators of success, such as quality of life. Reduction in leg volume usually occurs slowly, unless bandages are used. The largest reductions in leg volume tend to occur at the beginning of lymphoedema management. With time, the rate of volume reduction decreases, a trend that can be discouraging for some patients. For these and other reasons, we do not advise that volume reduction be considered a major indicator of the success in lymphoedema management.

Final Words

In this book, you have learned basic important information on how to manage lymphoedema in filariasis-endemic areas. Through the years of writing this book, we have had the sense of running in an ever-expanding relay race. The prize for the winning team will be the satisfaction and joy of eliminating lymphatic filariasis—not only the filarial worm, but the suffering experienced by millions of people who already have, or are at risk of, chronic lymphoedema. Now that you, a health worker in a filariasis-endemic area, have read this book, we pass the baton in this relay race to you. You can be a source of knowledge, new skills, and encouragement to your patients, and in turn, pass this baton of hope to them, their families, and their communities.

Recommended Reading

Dreyer G, Addiss D. Hope Clubs: new strategy for lymphatic filariasis-endemic areas. Bulletin of Tropical Medicine and International Health (Newsletter of Royal Society of Tropical Medicine and Hygiene). 2000; 8(1):8.

Dunyo SK. Scarification as a risk factor for rapid progression of filarial elephantiasis. *Trans Roy Soc Trop Med Hyg* 1997; 91:446.

Recommended Viewing

Lymphatic Filariasis: Hope For A Better Life. (Training video). Program for patients, 21 minutes. Program for health care workers, 58 minutes.

For further information on the scientific publications please contact a university or medical school library, or write to Centers for Disease Control and Prevention (contact information on page 111).

Copies of the video may be purchased through the Public Health Foundation in the United States (contact information on page 111).

INDIVIDUAL SHEET EVALUATION – ENTRY LESIONS

Name: Id: age: sex:

1. Lower limbs – interdigital entry lesions

		1st	2nd	3rd	4th	
Date:___ / ___ / ___	Left	☐	☐	☐	☐	Stage:

For example:
1st = between big toe and second toe

		1st	2nd	3rd	4th	
	Right	☐	☐	☐	☐	Stage:

Comments:_____

_____

2. Upper limbs – interdigital entry lesions

		1st	2nd	3rd	4th	
Date:___ / ___ / ___	Left	☐	☐	☐	☐	Stage:

For example:
1st = between thumb and forefinger

		1st	2nd	3rd	4th	
	Right	☐	☐	☐	☐	Stage:

Comments:_____

_____

3. Other lesions (including bottom of the folds)

Date:___ / ___ / ___

Anatomical location:_____

_____

Characteristics (type of secretion, size, shape, other)_____

_____

Duration / Potential cause: _____

_____

Proposed Treatment (Hygiene, antiseptics, creams, oral antibiotics, systemic antibiotics, elevation, exercises, cold compress, medicine for fever, rest, bandages)

_____

_____

HYGIENE EVALUATION

Date:____/____/____   Patient ID: _____

Visit: ☐ 1st   ☐ 2nd   ☐ 3rd   ☐ Routine

1. No Help is needed   ☐

2. **Help is needed**   ◼

    a. Help is Available   ☐   _____

        • Family   ☐ (Who?):   Same Residence? ☐ Yes ☐ No

        • Friend   ☐

        • Hope Club   ☐

    b. Help is Not Available ◼

3. Correct Hygiene   ☐

4. **Incorrect Hygiene**   ◼

      Areas in need of 1._____

        improvement: 2._____

                 3._____

                 4._____

                 5._____

                 6._____

    Proposed Solutions: _____

_____

_____

_____

5. Barriers: 1._____

               2._____

               3._____

               4._____

               5._____

               6._____

GLOSSARY

Acute attack: The signs and symptoms (including swelling, warmth, redness, and pain of the affected area, fever, chills, headache, and weakness) caused by a bacterial infection of the skin. Bacteria enter the body through entry lesions in the skin.

Adverse: Unintended, unwanted, undesirable. For example, people with many microfilariae in their blood may develop the adverse reactions of fever, headache, and body aches after treatment with DEC.

Adjunct measures: Treatment measures that may be helpful for some patients, but may not be necessary for others. For example, surgery to remove knobs may be a useful adjunct measure for people with stage 4 lymphoedema of the leg.

Amputation: Surgical removal, usually of the leg or arm.

Anterograde lymphangitis: Anterograde is a medical word that means "forwards", or moving away from the extremities towards the trunk or centre of the body. Lymphangitis is inflammation of the lymphatic vessels. In acute bacterial attacks, streaks of inflammation may sometimes be seen along the lymphatic vessels, moving away from the limbs towards trunk. See "retrograde lymphangitis".

Antibacterial cream: A cream that kills bacteria or stops them from growing. Antibacterial creams are used to treat infected entry lesions and wounds. They are also used to prevent infections in deep folds.

Antibiotic: A drug that is used to treat bacterial infections. Antibiotics are prescribed by a doctor. They can be given by mouth (tablets or pills) or by injection.

Antifilarial drug: A drug that kills microfilariae in the blood and may (or may not) kill adult worms in the lymphatic vessels. Antifilarial drugs are used to treat filarial infections.

Antifungal cream: A cream that kills fungi or stops them from growing. Antifungal creams are used to treat entry lesions between the toes. For patients with advanced stage lymphoedema, antifungal creams can help prevent fungal infections in the deep folds and in the interdigital spaces.

Antiseptic: Anything that stops or delays bacteria from growing. Antiseptics are used on the skin.

Aspirin: A medicine taken to reduce pain and fever. Aspirin is not usually recommended for people who live in areas where the disease dengue occurs.

Axilla: Armpit.

Bacteria: A type of germ that can enter the skin and cause acute attacks.

Bandages: Strips of cloth or other material used to compress the leg, reduce its volume, and collapse the venous varices near the surface of the skin.

Blood clot: A clot (a solid or soft lump) that forms in the veins, primarily in the legs, and usually in people with other diseases or those who have stayed in bed or without moving for long periods of time.

Brugia malayi: The filarial parasite that causes about 10% of lymphatic filariasis in the world. *Brugia malayi* is found in parts of Asia and the Western Pacific.

Capacity: Ability.

Chronic: Lasting a long time.

Chyluria: A condition in which the urine is white or milky in colour. The urine may also be pink or red if blood is present. Chyluria is caused by leaking of lymph fluid from damaged lymphatic vessels into the urine.

Clean water: Water that is suitable for drinking.

Clot: A soft or solid lump that can sometimes be found in the urine of patients with chyluria. See also "blood clot".

Cluster: Group, bunch.

Clustered: Grouped together, bunched.

Congenital: Existing at birth. People who have congenital lymphoedema are born with damaged or abnormal lymphatic vessels.

Contraindication: A reason not to give a certain medicine or do a specific medical procedure. For example, pregnancy is a contraindication to treatment with antifilarial drugs.

Cosmetic surgery: Surgery done to improve the way a person looks. Cosmetic surgery to remove knobs may also decrease the risk of entry lesions in some patients.

Debride: To remove dead tissue, as from a wound.

DEC: Diethylcarbamazine, an antifilarial drug. DEC kills microfilariae in the blood and some adult worms in the lymphatic vessels.

Deep skin fold: A skin fold in which the base or bottom can be seen only when the edges of the fold are separated by hand. Deep folds are a sign of advanced lymphoedema (at least stage 5). Because deep folds are often moist, fungi and bacteria grow easily there.

Definitive: final, certain.

Dengue: A disease that is transmitted by mosquitoes, and which causes fever, headache, body aches, and other symptoms, but not lymphoedema.

Diabetes: A disease in which there is too much sugar in the blood.

Diagnosis: The determination of the cause or nature of a disease

Diethylcarbamazine: See DEC.

Differential diagnosis: Determination of the diseases that could possibly explain the signs and symptoms in a particular patient

Dilate: To make wider or larger, to expand or swell.

Dilated: Stretched, distended, expanded, or enlarged.

Disability: Inability to adequately or independently perform routine daily activities such as walking, bathing, going to the bathroom, etc. Disabled patients need help from the health care system.

Drowsiness: Sleepiness.

Elderly: Old people.

Electron microscope: An instrument that can make very small objects, such as filarial worms, look very large.

Elephantiasis: Severe or advanced lymphoedema.

Elevation: Raising up. Elevation of the leg allows fluid to drain. People with lymphoedema of the leg should elevate their legs at night by raising the foot of the bed so that the heel of the patient's foot is above the level of the heart. Elevation is not harmful for normal legs without lymphoedema.

Elongated: Long in shape.

Endemic areas: Areas where a disease occurs or is well established.

Entry lesion: Any break in the skin that allows bacteria to enter the body. Entry lesions can occur between the toes or in deep folds. Wounds on the skin surface, such as cuts, scrapes, or scratches, are also entry lesions. Almost all patients with acute attacks will have visible entry lesions.

Epidemiologic: Related to epidemiology.

Epidemiology: The study of patterns, distribution, and occurrence of disease.

Exercise: Active movement of the muscles. Exercise helps move fluid away from the tissues. Exercise can be done anywhere and at any time, while sitting, lying, or standing. It is good to exercise as often as possible.

Exudate: Fluid that oozes or leaks from a wound.

Facilitate: To make easier, to assist.

Fat: An oily or greasy substance found in many foods.

Fatigue: Tiredness, lack of energy.

Fever: Abnormally high body temperature.

Filarial infection: The presence of adult filarial worms in the lymphatic vessels, or of microfilariae in the blood.

Filariasis: Lymphatic filariasis.

Flow: To move easily, as a liquid or a stream of water.

Fluid: Liquid.

Fold: A crease. As lymphoedema gets worse, the swelling and hardening of the skin often occur unevenly, more in some areas than in others. This causes a skin fold to appear. Skin folds can be shallow or deep. Shallow folds often become deep as the swelling increases.

Fungal infection: Infection with fungi.

Fungi: A type of germ that causes infections between the toes and is the most common cause of entry lesions. These entry lesions make it easier for bacteria to enter the skin and cause acute attacks. Fungi themselves do not cause acute attacks.

Fusiform: Elongated, spindle-shaped.

Genitals: Sex organs.

Germs: Small living organisms, such as fungi and bacteria, which can cause infections in humans. Germs can be seen only with a microscope.

Granulation tissue: New tissue that forms in healing wounds, ulcers, and other conditions, such as ingrown toenails.

Haematuria: Blood in the urine.

Heal: To make well or healthy again.

Health care system: Doctors, nurses, community health workers and other health care workers and resources.

Heart: The organ that pumps blood through the body.

Hydrocoele: Collection of too much fluid inside the scrotal sac, which causes the scrotum to swell or get larger.

Hygiene: Cleanliness. Hygiene involves washing with soap and water until the rinse water is clean, and then carefully drying.

Infected wounds: Wounds in which bacteria are present and are multiplying, causing disease.

Infection: The presence and growth in the body of any germ or organism that can cause disease.

Inflammation: The word "inflammation" means "in flames" and describes redness, pain, swelling and warmth. In patients with dark skin, the redness of inflammation may be hard to see. However, you can feel the warmth of the skin. Swelling is one of the signs of inflammation, but it can also be present without inflammation.

Inguinal: In or near the groin.

Insufficiency: Inadequacy, inability.

Interdigital: Between the toes (on the foot) or between the fingers (on the hand).

Intestine: Bowel.

Itch: An irritating feeling on the skin that creates the desire to scratch.

Ivermectin: A drug that kills microfilariae in the blood. Ivermectin also kills some worms that live in the intestines.

Keloid: A protruding scar.

Knobs: Small bumps, lumps or protrusions on the skin. Knobs in their natural state (before treatment) feel very firm, even hard. With treatment, knobs may become softer and smaller, and even disappear. Knobs are found in stage 4 lymphoedema or higher.

Leg volume: The size of the leg.

Limb: Leg or arm.

Lymph fluid (lymph): Fluid found in the lymphatic vessels. Lymph fluid is made up of water, waste products, and cells that fight bacteria. Lymph fluid can be white (when it contains fat), straw-coloured, or, if blood is present, reddish.

Lymph nodes (also called lymph glands): Small, bean-shaped organs along the lymphatic vessels. The lymph nodes trap bacteria before they reach the blood.

Lymph scrotum: A disease in which the scrotal sac is thick and enlarged, and has vesicles on the surface of the skin that are filled with (and frequently leak) lymph fluid.

Lymphatic filariasis: The disease caused by infection with filarial worms and the long-term results of this infection.

Lymphatic system: The network of vessels and lymph nodes that carries lymph fluid, bacteria, and waste products from the tissues. The lymphatic system helps fight infections.

Lymphatic vessels: A system of tubes that carry lymph fluid. Lymphatic vessels are similar to blood vessels, but instead of blood, they move fluid, waste products, and some bacteria away from the tissues and towards the heart. Adult filarial worms live in the lymphatic vessels.

Lymphoedema: Swelling caused by the collection of fluid in the tissue. Lymphoedema most frequently occurs in the legs, arm, breasts, scrotal skin, and penis.

Macerated: Moist and soft.

Malleolus: One of two rounded prominent bones on either side of the ankle.

Manage: To take care of; to treat.

Mass treatment: Giving a drug or medicine to all members of a community.

Medicated cream: Antibacterial or antifungal cream.

Medial malleolus: The rounded prominent bone on the inside of the ankle.

Microfilaria: A "baby" worm that is produced by the adult female worm in the lymphatic vessels. Microfilariae are found in the blood and are taken up by mosquitoes during a blood meal.

Microscope: An instrument that makes it possible to see very small things that cannot be seen with the naked eye (such as microfilariae and bacteria).

Mimic: Imitate.

Moist: Wet or damp.

Mossy lesions: Clusters of vesicles that look like moss, or warts, or the head of a cauliflower. Mossy lesions usually occur on the foot, where they are known as "mossy foot". The presence of mossy lesions is the feature of stage 6 lymphoedema.

Myiasis: A disease caused by flies laying their eggs in wounds or in entry lesions.

Nodule: A lump.

Oedema (or edema): Swelling. Oedema is caused by excess fluid in the tissue. Oedema can occur with or without inflammation.

Onychomycosis: fungal infection of the nails.

Paracetomol: A medicine that reduces fever and pain.

Parasite: An animal that lives in, or on, another animal (known as the host), and which may harm the host. The filarial worms *Wuchereria bancrofti* and *Brugia malayi* are parasites of humans.

Parasitic worms: Worms that live in the human body. Filarial worms are one type of parasitic worms.

Penis: The male sex and urinary organ.

Permeable: Allowing air or water to pass through.

Physical examination: Touching and looking at a patient to diagnose his or her health problem.

Pigmented: Coloured.

Plaque: A raised area or patch.

Potassium permanganate: A type of antiseptic that is used on wounds, in interdigital spaces, and on deep folds. Potassium permanganate is poured over the skin to help fight bacterial infections. It comes in the form of a purple tablet or powder. It must be mixed well with clean water.

Prognosis: Prediction or forecast of how much and how quickly the patient's condition will improve or get worse.

Prophylactic antibiotics: Antibiotics given to prevent bacterial infections. Prophylactic antibiotics are prescribed by a doctor when the patient continues to have acute attacks in spite of other measures. They are usually given by injection, but they can be given by mouth. People with advanced lymphoedema often need prophylactic antibiotics.

Protein: A substance in food, found particularly in meat, that helps build strong bodies.

Psoriasis: A disease characterized by patches of red, scaly skin.

Pulmonary embolism: A serious medical condition in which a blood clot in a vein is loosened and travels to the lungs, where it blocks the flow of blood to the lungs.

Pus: The yellow-white or greenish material that is produced by, and often drains from, an infection.

Reconstructive surgery: Surgery to "reconstruct" or "rebuild" part of the body.

Repeated acute attacks: Acute attacks that occur again and again.

Retrograde lymphangitis: Retrograde is a medical word that means "backwards", or moving towards the fingers or toes. Lymphangitis is inflammation of the lymphatic vessels. When the adult worm dies, streaks of inflammation can be seen along the lymphatic vessels, moving down the body towards the foot or hand. This is known as retrograde lymphangitis. See "anterograde lymphangitis".

Reversible swelling: Swelling that goes away, or comes and goes.

Risk factor: Something that increases risk. For example, in people who have lymphoedema, poor hygiene and poor skin care are risk factors for acute attacks.

Rotate: To move in a circle.

Scratch: To scrape or rub, especially with the fingernails.

Scrotal: Of the scrotum.

Scrotal sac: Scrotum. The sac or pouch of skin, located beneath the penis, which holds the testicles.

Scrotum: The sac of skin, located beneath the penis, which holds the testicles.

Self-confidence: Belief or trust in oneself or one's own abilities.

Self-esteem: Self-confidence.

Shallow skin fold: A skin fold in which the base is visible when the leg or arm moves so that the fold "opens". If a patient has a shallow fold at the ankle, the base of the fold can be seen when he or she points the toes downwards. Shallow folds occur in persons with stage 3 lymphoedema or higher.

Skin: The outer covering of the body.

Spontaneously: Happening without obvious or known cause. For example, adult filarial worms may die spontaneously, without antifilarial treatment.

Stage: The degree of severity of lymphoedema. Lymphoedema is graded from stage 1 (mild) to stage 7 (very severe).

Stage 1 lymphoedema: Swelling is reversible overnight.

Stage 2 lymphoedema: Swelling is not reversible overnight.

Stage 3 lymphoedema: One or more shallow skin folds are present.

Stage 4 lymphoedema: One or more knobs are present.

Stage 5 lymphoedema: One or more deep skin folds are present.

Stage 6 lymphoedema: Mossy lesions are present.

Stage 7 lymphoedema: The patient is unable to adequately or independently perform routine daily activities such as walking, bathing, cooking, etc. He or she needs help from health care system.

Steroid: A type of medicine that reduces inflammation. Steroid cream is sometimes used to reduce inflammation in entry lesions.

Streaking: The appearance of an inflamed lymphatic vessel, which looks like a "streak" or cord that is red, tender, and warm. Adult worm death causes retrograde streaking and bacterial infection causes anterograde streaking.

Subcutaneous: Under the skin.

Suffocate: To die from lack of air; smother.

Swell: To increase in volume or size.

Systemic antibiotics (see antibiotics): Antibiotics that are given by injection or by mouth.

Tender: Sensitive or painful when touched.

Testicles: Male sex organs (testes).

Tissue: A group of similar cells in the body. Muscles and skin are two examples of tissues.

Topical: On the skin. Topical antibiotics are applied to the skin, in a cream, for example.

Torsion of the testes (testicular torsion): Abnormal twisting or rotation of the testes, resulting in a lack of blood and severe pain, which threatens the capacity of the testis to remain alive.

Translucent: Partially transparent; allowing some light to pass through.

Transparent: Clear, allowing light to pass through.

Trauma: Injury or hurt, usually occurring suddenly.

Traumatized: Injured.

Urinary tract: The organs involved in making and releasing urine from the body.

Urogenital: Related to the sex or urinary organs.

Varicose veins: Enlarged, twisted veins that result from venous disease.

Venous insufficiency: A condition in which the veins do not have the ability or capacity to return blood to the heart as well as they should.

Vesicle: A blister. A small elevated area of skin that contains fluid.

Vicious cycle: A situation in which one problem leads to another problem, which in turn, makes the first problem worse, and so on.

Worm: A long soft-bodied animal. Intestinal worms live in the intestines, while adult filarial worms live in the lymphatic vessels.

Wounds: Cuts, scrapes, or scratches in the skin caused by injury. Wounds are one type of entry lesion, usually on the surface of the skin. Entry lesions may also be caused by fungal infections between the toes or in skin folds. For the purposes of this book, that type of interdigital entry lesion is not considered to be a wound.

Wuchereria bancrofti: The filarial parasite that causes 90% of lymphatic filariasis in the world. *Wuchereria bancrofti* is found in Asia, Africa, the Pacific Islands, and the Americas.

INDEX

A

Acute attacks, Ch. 5
  Alcoholics, special attention necessary for, 50
  Antibiotics, use of, 49–50, 62
  Antiseptics, lessening occurrence of through use of, 43
  Aspirin, management with, cautions, 49
  Assessment of, 47–48
  Bacterial infection as cause of, 9, 61–62, 73
  Chronic disease sufferers, special attention necessary for, 50
  Danger signs, 50
  Diabetics as needing special attention, 50
  Drowsiness during as danger sign, 50
  Elderly persons, 50
  Entry lesions, hygiene and treatment of, 49, 62
  Exercise during, 39–41, 49
  Fever as symptom of, 47, 50, 62
  Frequency of as indication of treatment success, 52, 85
  Harmful practices, 50–51
  Inflammation as sign of, 47
  Inguinal area, first site of, 47
  Liquids, importance of, 49
  Malnourished patients, special attention necessary for, 50
  Pain relief, 48–49
    cooling measures, 48–49
    medicine for fever, 49
    rest and elevations measures, 49
  Paracetomol, use as treatment during, 49
  Penis, effect of on, 9, 61
  Pregnant women, special attention necessary for, 50
  Publications of interest, list of, 52
  Scrotum, 61
  Tips for management of, 51
  Training video, details about, 52
Adverse drug reactions, 3–5
  Fatigue, 3
  Fever, 3
Adjunct measures, 42–44, 60
  Antibiotics, 60
  Bandaging as, 42–43
  Breathing exercises, 43
  Compressive measures, 42–43
  Cosmetic surgery, 44
  Emollients, 42
  Massage, 43
  Pregnancy, during, 71–72
  Prophylactic antibiotics, 43–44
  Urogenital problems, for, 60
  Stockings, 43
Albendazole, 3
Alcoholics, acute attacks in, special care needed, 50
Amputation, 69, 76, 83
  Antibiotics, necessity of, 83
  Diabetes, due to, 69
  Mycetoma, due to, 76
Anterograde lymphangitis, 47
Antibacterial cream, 31–34, 59
Antibiotics
  Acute attack management, 49–50, 62
  Adjunct measure, as, 60
  Amputation and, 83
  Bacterial infection treated with, 43–44
  Prophylactic, 43–44, 60, 83
  Systemic antibiotics, 49, 50
Antifilarial drugs, ii
  Contraindications, 5
  Hope clubs, distribution of by, 83
  Hydrocoele and, 53

Limitations of, 23
Mass treatment with, 5
Microfilariae in blood, 4–5
Pregnancy and, 4
Antifungal cream, 32, 35
Diabetes and, 35, 69
Hydrocoele management and, 55
Antiseptics
Acute attacks, lessening of with use of, 43
Debriding, recommendation against
using for, 31
Entry lesion management with, 29–31, 49
Genitals, use of on, 60
Hygiene and skin care with, 34
Aspirin
Acute attack management with,
cautions, 49
Dengue, not recommended in areas of,
49
Assessment of chronic lymphoedema,
Ch. 3
See also Acute attacks
Stage 1, 15–16
Stage 2, 17
Stage 3, 17
Stage 4, 17–19
Stage 5, 19
Stage 6, 19
Stage 7, 21
Staging features, overview, 13–15, 21
Training video, information on, 22
Axilla, lymph nodes in, removal of, 73

B

Bacteria
Acute attacks caused by bacterial infec-
tion, 9, 61–62, 73
Antibacterial creams, 31–34
Antibiotics and, 43–44
Chromoblastomycosis and, 76
Dressing, occlusive and semi-occlusive, 72
Entry lesions and, 8–9, 27, 29, 47
Fever as indication of infection, 33

Hygiene as method of reducing, 9, 23
Inflammation caused by, 9, 47
Infections, effect of lymphatic filariasis, i
Lymphatic system, destruction of by,
7–9
Mossy lesions and, 19
Scrotum, bacterial infection of, 62
Severe oedema of penis and, 60
Wounds infected by, tips for recogniz-
ing, 33
Bandages
Adjunct measure, as, 42
Entry lesions, use of on, 43
Incorrect use of, effects, 42
Inflammation, use of during, 42
Itching caused by, 42
Leg volume reduction through use of, 87
Occlusive and semi-occlusive, bacterial
infection and, 72
Self-care and, 80
Blisters and entry lesions, 41
Blood clot, bed confinement, lengthy,
danger of, 21
Blood, microfilariae in, antifilarial drug
treatment, 4–5
Breasts, swelling of, differential diagnosis, 75
Breathing exercises, 43
Brugia malayi, percentage of infections
caused by, 2

C

Capacity
Lymphatic filariasis, effect of on, i
Lymphatic insufficiency, 7
Veins, reduced, 67
Children
Education of about disease, 80
Endemic areas, special dangers for, 80
Hydrocoele and, 75
Lymph nodes chiefly affected by dis-
ease, 10
Vesicles, 73
Wuchereria bancrofti, site of in, 10

Chromoblastomycosis, causes of, 76
Chronic lymphoedema, assessment of, see
    Assessment of chronic lymphoedema
Chyluria, 10, 63–65
    Diabetes and, 77
    Effects of, 63–64
    Fat intake reduction as management
        tool, 64, 77
    Fever, 63
    Management of, 64–65
Community resources for management of
    disease, 84
Community treatment for, Ch. 1
    Antifilarial drugs, 5
    DEC-fortified salt, 3
    Publications of interest, list of, 5–6
Complications, management in endemic
    areas, Ch. 7
    Diabetes, 69
    Leprosy, 70–71
    Myiasis, 71
    Occlusive and semi-occlusive dressings,
        72
    Pregnancy, 71–72
    Psoriasis, 70
    Publications of interest, list of, 72
    Veins, diseases of, 67–69
    Venous insufficiency, 67–69
    Venous ulcer, 67–69
Compressive measures, exercise, use of
    makes easier, 43
Congenital abnormalities, 73, 75
Contraindications, antifilarial drug treat-
    ment, 5
Cosmetic surgery, 44
    Knob removal by, 44
Counselling, use of for men with urogeni-
    tal problems, 60

D
—

Debriding, antiseptics, not recommended
    for, 31
Deep skin fold

Emollients, not recommended, 42
Entry lesion site, 29
    Hygiene for, 35–36
    Stage 5 lymphoedema, main feature of,
        19
    Potassium permanganate, used in, 31
    Staging feature, as, 13
Definitions, 91
Dengue, aspirin not recommended in
    areas of, 49
Diabetes, 69
    Acute attacks and sufferers of, 50
    Amputation, 69
    Antifungal cream and, 35, 69
    Entry lesions and, 69
    Milky urine, 77
    Risk factor, as, 34
Diagnosis, differential, Ch. 8
    Inguinal hernia, 77
    Knobs, 76
    Lipedema, 75
    Milky urine, 77
    Publications of interest, list of, 78
    Swelling
        breasts, 75
        genitals, 75
        limbs, 73
Diethylcarbamazine (DEC), 3
    Adverse reactions, 5
    Salt fortified with as treatment, 3
Dressing, see Bandages
Drowsiness, acute attack, during, as dan-
    ger sign, 50

E
—

Eczema, symptoms of, 69
Edema, see Oedema
Education of patients about disease, 80
Elderly persons, acute attack and, special
    treatment needed, 50
Elephantiasis
    Knobs as indication of, 57
    Scrotum and penis, 57, 59–60

Elevation, 37–39
    Cautions regarding, 39
    Importance of, 37
    Lying down, 39
    Sitting, 37
Emollients
    Endemic areas, use of not recom-
        mended, 42
    Deep skin folds and, 42
    Mossy lesions, use of not recom-
        mended, 42
Endemic areas
    Children in, 80
    Drug donations to, GlaxoSmithKline, 3
    Emollients, use not recommended, 42
    Hydrocoele in, 55
    Hygiene in, importance of, 36
    Keloids (knobs) common in, 17
    Legs as most common site infection, 15
    Management complications of, Ch. 7
Entry lesion, see Lesions
Exercise
    Acute attacks and, 39, 49
    Breathing, 43
    Circle exercise, 41
    Compressive measures conducive to, 43
    Excess water removed from tissues by, 7
    Management tool, as, 23
    Not recommended in certain circum-
        stances, 60
    Specific beneficial exercises described,
        39–41
    Toe point exercise, 39–41
    Up on the toes exercise, 39
Exudate
    Eczema, occasional characteristic of, 69
    Increase in as indication of infection, 33

F
—

Fat
    Chyluria
        as cause of colour of, 63
        reducing fat intake for manage-
    ment of, 64, 77

Fatigue, adverse drug reaction, 3
Fever
    Acute attack, symptom of, 47, 50
    Adverse drug reaction, 3
    Bacterial infection, indication of, 33
    Chyluria and, 63
    Psoriasis and, 70
Folds, see particular type, e.g., deep skin
    fold
Fungal infection
    Chromoblastomycosis, 76
    Entry lesions caused by, 29
    Hydrocoeles and, 55
    Hygiene for, 25, 35–36
    Itching as sign of, 32
    Occlusive and semi-occlusive dressings
        and, 72
    Recognizing, tips for, 33
    Scrotum, 53
    Staging feature, use as, 15
    Treatment of, 32
Fungi
    Chromoblastomycosis caused by, 76
    Entry lesions, as cause of, 29
    Mycetoma caused by, 76

G
—

Genitals, Ch. 6
    See also specific sex organs
    Entry lesions, 59
    Other diseases as cause of swelling and
        disfigurement, 73
    Swelling of, differential diagnosis, 75
GlaxoSmithKline, donation of drugs in
    endemic areas, 3
Glossary, 91

H
—

Haematuria, 63
Hope clubs, 81–83
    Antifilarial drug distribution through, 83

Hydrocoele, 53–62
    Antifilarial drugs and, 55
    Antifungal cream, as management tool,
    55
    Children and, 75
    Diagnosis, difficulty of, 73
    Endemic areas, levels of in, 55
    Fungal infections and, 55
    Inguinal hernia mistaken for, 77
    Management of, 55–56
    Nonhereditary nature of, 3
Hygiene, 25–29
    Bacterial infection control by, 9, 23, 27
    Deep skin folds, 35–36
    Endemic areas, importance, 36
    Evaluation sheet for, 90
    Fungal infections, 27, 35–36
    Illustration of steps of, 24–25
    Lymph scrotum, 62
    Management tool, as, 25–29
    Penis, 59, 62
    Scrotum, 62
    Steroids used for, 35
    Tips on, 35–37
    Washing, 25–29
        drying afterward, 29
        examination of skin, 27
        legs, step-by-step guide, 27
        supplies necessary, 27

I
—

Inflammation
    Acute attack, as sign of, 47
    Bacteria as cause of, 8, 47
    Bandages and, 43
    Response to death of adult worm, as, 4
    Signs of, 4
    Spread of, 4
Inguinal area
    Hernia, 77
    Site of first sign of acute attack, 47
Intestine
    Albendazole as drug to kill worms in, 3

Inguinal hernia of, 77
Itching
    Bandages as cause of, 42
    Eczema, characteristic of, 69
    Fungal infection, sign of, 33
    Psoriasis, effect of, 70
    Venous ulcers, common effect of, 69
Ivermectin, 3

K
—

Keloids, 76
    Endemic areas, common in, 17
    Stage 4 feature of lymphoedema, 17
Knobs, 76
    Cosmetic surgery for removal of, 44
    Elephantiasis, as indication of, 57
    Leprosy and, 70–71
    Mossy lesions and, distinguishing
    between, 19
    Stage 4 feature of lymphoedema, 17
    Staging feature, as, 13
    Varicose buttons as, 19

L
—

Leg volume
    Bandages, reduction through use of, 87
    Increase of at higher stages of disease,
    15
    Monitoring of as indication of success-
    ful treatment, 87
Leprosy, 70–71
    Knobs and, 70–71
Lesions
    Entry
        antibacterial cream for, 33
        antibiotics, prophylactic, for
        severe lesions, 43–44
        antiseptics as management tool
        for, 29–31, 49
        bacteria and, 8–9, 27, 29, 47
        bandages and, 43

blisters and, 41
deep skin fold as place of, 29
definition of, 8
diabetes and, 69
evaluation sheet for, 89
flies attracted to, danger of, 36
fungal infection as cause of, 29
fungi as cause of, 29
hygiene and, 9, 23, 27, 36, 49
ice, use of not recommended, 34
illustrations of, 14
lipedema and, 75
lymphoedema feature, 16–21
management of, 29–34
medicated creams for, 31–34
multiple sites of possible, 15
myiasis and, 71
shoes and, 23
venous insufficiency and, 69
Mossy
bacterial infection and, 19
chromoblastomycosis, differenti
ating from, 76
emollients, not recommended
for, 42
knobs, distinguishing between,
19
stage 6 lymphoedema feature, 19
staging feature, as, 13
Limbs, swelling of, differential diagnosis,
73
Lipedema, 75
Lymphatic insufficiency, 7
Lymphatic vessels, filariasis and, Ch. 2
Adult worms, damage caused by, 8
Children, 10
Damaged vessels
draining sites other than skin,
consequences, 10
draining skin, consequences of,
8–9
Lymphatic system overview, 7–8
Publications of interest, list of, 11–12
Lymph fluid
Definition of, 7
Flow of changed as symptom of dis-

ease, 8–9
Lymph nodes (lymph glands), 7
Bacteria destruction as function of, 7
Children, filariasis and, 10
Locations of, 8
Removal of, effects, 73
Lymphoedema programs, achieving,
maintaining, monitoring of, Ch. 9
Lymphoedema stages, see Stages of lym-
phoedema
Lymph scrotum, 57–59
Hygiene, importance of, 62
Management of, 59–60
Prophylactic antibiotics for, 60
Surgery, 60

M

Malleolus, 69
Malnourished patients, acute attacks in,
special attention necessary, 50
Management of lymphoedema, Ch. 4, Ch.
7
See also Acute attacks
Adjunct measures, 42–44
bandages, 42–43
breathing exercises, 43
compressive measures, 42–43
cosmetic surgery, 44
emollients, 42
massage, 43
prophylactic antibiotics, 43–44
Basic components of, 23
Community resources, 84
Complications, endemic areas, Ch. 7
Elevation, 37–39
lying down, 39
sitting, 37
Entry lesions, 29–34
antibacterial creams, 33–34
antifungal creams, 33
antiseptics, 29–31
medicated creams, 31–32
potassium permanganate, 31

Exercise, 23, 39–41
    breathing, 43
    circle exercise, 41
    toe point, 39–41
    up on the toes, 39
Generally, Ch. 4, 44
Hygiene, 25–29, 34–37
    drying, 29
    skin examination, 27
    supplies needed, 27
    wash affected leg, 27
Need for, 23
Patient management plan, 45
Publications of interest, list of, 45–46
Shoes, 41
Skin care, tips for, 34–37
Steps in, 25–45
Training video, details about, 46
Massage, 43
Medial malleolus, 67
Microfilaria, 1
    Annual treatment for necessary, 3
    Blood, in, see Blood, microfilaria in
    Drugs effective against, 3, 4–5
    Mosquitoes, development of within, 1
Milky urine
    See also Chyluria
    Differential diagnosis, 77
Mossy legions, see Legions
Mycetoma, fungi as cause of, 76
Myiasis, 71
    Entry lesions and, 71
    Occlusive and semi-occlusive dressings,
    use of in treatment of, 72

O

Occlusive and semi-occlusive dressings, 72
    Bacterial infection and, 72
    Entry lesions and, 72
    Fungal infections and, 72
    Myiasis and, 72
    Psoriasis and, 72
Oedema (edema)

Penis, severe, 60
Pregnancy, during, 71–72
Onychomycosis
    Nail trimming in case of, 27
    Staging feature, use of as, 15

P

Paracetomol, acute attacks, use in treating,
    49
Patient management plan, development
    of, 45
Penis
    See also Genitals; Urogenital problems
    in filariasis
    Acute attacks, effect of repeated on, 9,
    61–62
    Antiseptics, use of on discouraged, 90
    Bacterial infections of, 60
    Condoms, cautions on use of, 60
    Elephantiasis and, 57, 60
    Exercise, 60
    Hygiene, importance of, 59, 62
    Lymph scrotum and, 57
    Oedema of, 60–61
    Skin of, problems affecting, 57–62
        acute attacks, 61–62
        counselling, 60
        elephantiasis, 57
        lymphoedema, 57
        lymph scrotum, 57–59
        management of, 59–60
        prophylactic antibiotics, 60
        pubic hair, 60
        severe oedema of penis, 60–61
        sexually transmitted diseases,
        prevention of, 60
        surgery, 60
    Surgery on, 60
Potassium permanganate
    Antiseptic, use as, 29
    Deep skin fold, use of in, 31
    Safety of, 31
Pregnancy, 71–72

Acute attacks and, special treatment
necessary, 50
Adjunct measures during, 71–72
Antifilarial drugs and, 4
Oedema during, 71–72
Venous insufficiency, 71–72
Programs, lymphoedema, achieving,
maintaining, monitoring of, Ch. 9
Benefits of, 84–85
Challenges, 83
    amputation, 83
    undesirable effects of programs, 83
Community resources, 84
Hope clubs, 81–83
Monitoring success
    leg volume as indicator, 87
    list of suggested indicators, 85–87
Publications of interest, list of, 87
Success
    achieving, 79–80
    benefits of, 84–85
    maintaining, 81
    monitoring, 85–87
Training video, details about, 87
Undesirable effects, 83
Prophylactic antibiotics, see Antibiotics
Psoriasis, 70
Fever and, 70
Itching as symptom of, 70
Occlusive or semi-occlusive dressings
used in treatment of, 72
Pubic hair, care of in case of urogenital
problems, 60
Pulmonary embolism, 21

S
—

Scrotum
See also Genitals; Hydrocoele; Urogeni-
tal problems in filariasis
Acute attacks in, 61–62
Antiseptics, use of on discouraged, 60
Bacterial infection of, 62
Exercise, 60

Fever as indication of acute attack in, 61
Fungal infections of, 55
Hygiene, importance of, 62
Lymph scrotum, 57–59
    hygiene, importance of, 62
    management of, 59–60
    prophylactic antibiotics for, 60
    surgery, 60
Skin problems of, 57–62
    acute attacks, 61–62
    counselling, 60
    elephantiasis, 57
    lymphoedema, 57
    lymph scrotum, 57–59
    management of, 59–60
    prophylactic antibiotics, 60
    pubic hair, 60
    severe oedema of penis, 60–61
    sexually transmitted diseases, `
    prevention of, 60
    surgery, 60
Self-care
Bandages, 80
Responsibility for, 79–80
Sexually transmitted diseases, prevention
of in case of urogenital problems, 60
Shallow skin fold
Stage 3 lymphoedema feature, 17
Staging feature, as, 13
Shoes, types of that are best for patients,
41
Skin
Care, tips for, 34–37
Condition, as indication of success of
program, 87
Stages of lymphoedema
Overview of, ii
Stage 1, 13, 15–16, 21, 45
Stage 2, 17, 21, 45
Stage 3, 15, 17, 21, 45
Stage 4, 13, 17–19, 21, 45
Stage 5, 19, 21, 45
Stage 6, 13, 15, 19, 21, 36, 44, 45
Stage 7, 13, 21, 45, 79
Steroids, hygiene, use in, 35
Stockings, as compressive measure, 43

Surgery
    Cosmetic, 44
    Urogenital problems, 60
Swelling, differential diagnosis
    Breasts, 75
    Genitals, 75
    Limbs, 73
Systemic antibiotics, see Antibiotics

T

Testicles, 8, 55
    See also Genitals; Hydrocoele; Urogenital problems in filariasis
    Testicular torsion, 62
Treatment, community, Ch. 1
    Drugs available for, 3, 4–5
        adverse reactions to, 3–4
    Elimination of lymphatic filariasis, WHO program for, 3
    Microfiariae in blood, medication for, 4–5

U

Urinary tract problems
    Chyluria, 63–65
    Haematuria, 63
    Milky urine, see Chyluria
Urogenital problems in filariasis, Ch. 6
    Genital problems, 53
    Hydrocoele, 53
    Publications of interest, list of, 66
    Scrotum and penis, skin problems, 57–62
        acute attacks, 61–62
        counselling, 60
        elephantiasis, 57
        lymphoedema, 57
        lymph scrotum, 57–59
        management of, 59–60
        prophylactic antibiotics, 60
        pubic hair, 60

    severe oedema of penis, 60–61
    sexually transmitted diseases, prevention of, 60
    surgery, 60
Urinary tract problems, 63–65
    chyluria, 63–65
    haematuria, 63

V

Varicose buttons, 19
Varicose veins, 67
Venous insufficiency, 19, 67–69
    Elevation of legs, importance of, 37
    Entry lesions, 69
    Pregnancy and, 71–72
    Staging feature, use of as, 15
Venous ulcers, 67–69
    Itching as common effect of, 69
Vesicles
    Children and, 73
    Lymph scrotum, 57, 59

W

Wuchereria bancrofti
    Children, site of in, 10
    Percentage of infections caused by, 2

RESOURCE INFORMATION

Additional information on lymphatic filariasis and lymphoedema management in filariasis-endemic areas is available from the following sources.

Copies of the "Hope Club Booklet" and some of the recommended reading materials mentioned in this book are available from:

> Centers for Disease Control and Prevention
> Division of Parasitic Diseases, Mailstop F-22
> Lymphatic Filariasis Unit
> 4770 Buford Highway, N.E.
> Atlanta, GA 30341
> USA
> Telephone: (1) 770-488-7760
> Fax: 770-488-7761

Copies of the videotape recommended in this book are available from:

> Public Health Foundation
> 1220 L Street, N.W. Suite 350
> Washington, D.C. 20005
> USA
> Telephone: (1) 202-898-5600
> Fax: 202-898-5609
>
> To order the videotape, call (1) 877-252-1200 or visit the online bookstore at *www.phf.org.*

Additional copies of this book are available from:

> Hollis Publishing Company
> 95 Runnells Bridge Road
> Hollis, New Hampshire 03049
> USA
> Telephone: 603-889-4500
> Fax: 603-889-6551
> Email: books@hollispublishing.com or visit the website at *www.hollispublishing.com*

Information on the Global Program to Eliminate Lymphatic Filariasis is available from:

The World Health Organization
20 Avenue Appia
1211 Geneva 27, Switzerland
Website: *www.filariasis.org*

The authors welcome your comments on this book and your suggestions for revisions in subsequent editions. Please contact:

Dr. Gerusa Dreyer
NGO Amaury Coutinho
Av Santos Dumont 333, Apt 1501
Aflitos
Recife, PE 52050-050
Brazil

Telephone: 55-81-3241-8807
Fax: 55-81-3242-7307
Email: gd@nlink.com.br

Dr. David Addiss
Centers for Disease Control and
Prevention
Division of Parasitic Diseases,
Mailstop F-22
Lymphatic Filariasis Unit
4770 Buford Highway, N.E.
Atlanta, GA 30341
USA

Telephone (1)-770-488-7760
Fax: (1)-770-488-7761
Email: daddiss@cdc.gov